MW00986578

Praise for *This Book Won't Make You Happy:
Eight Keys to Finding True Contentment*

"This book grabbed me from the very beginning. It is thought-provoking, insightful, full of practical tidbits, and a fun read."
—**Dr. Leah Katz**, psychologist and author of *Gutsy:
Mindfulness Practices for Everyday Bravery*

"A refreshingly novel twist on how to find happiness, based not on what happens in your life but how you relate to it. I'd highly recommend this book to anyone trying to find more ease and contentment in their daily life."
—**Dr. Kristin Neff**, author of *Self Compassion: The
Proven Power of Being Kind To Yourself* and associate
professor at University of Texas at Austin

"While this book might not make us happy, it does give us a path to what we need even more, contentment. Niro Feliciano writes with laugh-out-loud and relatable humor, honesty, intellect, and practical wisdom. She challenges our desire for a 'normal' life, and instead invites us to a life of health and wholeness. This book is a welcoming and timely guide to a life worth living."
—**Amy Julia Becker**, speaker and award-winning author of many
books, including *To Be Made Well* and *A Good and Perfect Gift*

"Niro Feliciano's work is relatable and compelling. She's a busy mom going in four separate directions, a wife who loves her husband, a friend who lends a listening ear, and a therapist who puts patients' needs first. I appreciate her humor and grace, and cherish the space she gives us in this book to share her insights."

—**Dr. Katie Takayasu**, physician, speaker, and author of *Plants First*

"Niro Feliciano is a down-to-earth authority on how we can best care for our mental well-being. Genuinely invested in supporting everyone facing unprecedented levels of anxiety and stress, Feliciano has a relatable, soothing, and valuable voice. Anyone seeking more contentment would benefit from her personal wisdom and research-based methods."

—**Maressa Brown**, journalist, author, and contributor to Parents.com

"Any conversation with Niro Feliciano is refreshing, challenging, and transformative. Her style of speaking and engagement transfers beautifully to the written word. Not only will you see yourself in her heartwarming and honest stories; you will begin to find a pathway to living with contentment."

—**Brenda Thorn**, J.D., executive pastor and care director, Hillsong East Coast

"One of the great new voices to emerge in our cultural crisis of anxiety is Niro Feliciano. There is nothing more elusive in our agitated culture than contentment. We all want it. In *This Book Won't Make You Happy*, Feliciano clears the path and walks you directly to it."

—**Rob Strong**, pastor and author of *The Big Guy Upstairs: You, Him, and How It All Works*

THIS BOOK
WON'T MAKE
YOU HAPPY

THIS BOOK won't make you Happy

EIGHT KEYS TO FINDING TRUE CONTENTMENT

NIRO FELICIANO, LCSW

BROADLEAF BOOKS
MINNEAPOLIS

THIS BOOK WON'T MAKE YOU HAPPY
Eight Keys to Finding True Contentment

The stories in this book reflect the author's recollection of events. Some names have been changed to protect the privacy of those depicted.

Cover design: Sydney Prusso

Print ISBN: 978-1-5064-8041-1
eBook ISBN: 978-1-5064-8042-8

To my Puerto-Lankan tribe,
Ed, Natalia, Samuel, Sofia, and Carolina:

This book didn't always make you happy, but
it never stopped you from cheering me on.
Thank you for being the reason I want what I've got.
With all my heart—this is for you.

Contents

Preface

"I don't know what's going on, but if something doesn't change, I don't think I'll make it. I don't think *we* will make it."

It was our sixteenth anniversary. Two successful careers; four beautiful, healthy kids; and a stunning home in an idyllic Connecticut suburb. Ours was the life people dreamed of . . . at least on the outside.

I looked across the candlelit table at my husband. Arms folded across my chest, I didn't want to be there. As far I was concerned, there was nothing to celebrate. Sitting across from him at our favorite restaurant, I didn't have much to say. The noise of other people's conversations echoing in the room filled the void created by our silence.

Then he spoke those words. He sounded angry, but I knew there was more underneath. As a therapist, I know the sound of desperation. I just never expected to hear it that day. I looked up from the floor into his eyes for the first time in weeks, maybe months. Sky blue and clear, his eyes were one of the first things I noticed about him when we met at an anti–Valentine's Day party in New York City nearly two decades ago. Yet now I saw deep pools of sadness. He looked like he had lost something that he wasn't sure he could get back.

He wasn't talking about divorce. We have never questioned our love and commitment to each other. In some ways, this was far worse. He was talking about survival—physical, emotional, and mental—all of which had been tested in both of us over the past several years and left us fractured and fragile.

I was angry. I felt misunderstood and unappreciated. From the moment I woke up in the morning, I hit the ground running, trying to get as much done as possible for as many people as possible. I knew he felt the same, rushing all day and night from one commitment to the next. Of course we both felt disconnected! When did we have time to connect—with anyone? This was the coveted, enchanted, "happy" life we created—and it was suffocating us both.

I finally spoke: "Do you know, once in a while, I think about what it would be like if I just disappeared? How much easier that would be . . ." My voice wavered for a moment as I looked away. As soon as the words came out, I couldn't believe I said them. I love my family, so why did these thoughts come and go so often recently? What had happened? How did we get here?

Ed paused for a moment, silent. Then he said quietly, "I have thought the same exact thing."

And that was the moment everything changed.

If this was the price of our so-called happiness, we were no longer willing to pay it.

I decided that night that we would never feel that way again.

And I never want you to either.

PART I

Why Is Happiness So Hard to Find?

CHAPTER 1

Normal

Once upon a time, before our world shape-shifted—when masks only appeared on Halloween night and no one thought twice about squeezing into packed venues, before screen time became a parent's worst enemy and before science morphed into politics—I wanted to write a book about happiness.

As a therapist, I had seen happiness become increasingly elusive to my clients. Year after year, over the last decade and a half in my office, I had started to see more and more people—and younger and younger ones—searching for it. Anxiety was at an all-time high. People were having a *really hard* time feeling good about their lives up against the constant backdrop of social media–curated perfection. Filtered pictures of friends on white, sandy Caribbean beaches, moms of three looking amazing in gray camo athleisure, and perfectly accessorized Pinterest-worthy living rooms all left people feeling like their lives didn't measure up. I heard clients constantly express, "I'm not good enough," "I don't have enough," or "I'm not smart or pretty or organized enough." I saw people constantly chasing what they thought they were supposed to be chasing—not only for themselves but for their kids—leaving them disconnected and exhausted, practically unable to enjoy anything that they had actually worked for. That's when I *really* wanted to write a book on happiness.

Even as thousands of books were published on the subject, I wondered why our rates of anxiety and depression continued to grow. Researchers had gotten into the happiness game as well. Studies, polls, and a plethora of pop culture articles all pointed to clear evidence as to what worked to improve our mood and, as important, what didn't. As therapists, we clearly had all the information we needed on how people could get happy. Then why weren't they?

Initially, I wanted to write a book to give you a list of simple things you could do to be happy. I wanted you to face your fears, try new things, dare to dream, and get excited about life. Like so many other authors had successfully done, I would send you on your way armed with a toolbox of helpful tips guaranteed to change your life for the better.

Then 2020 happened.

An unprecedented global pandemic. Lockdowns. School closures. Zoom everything. Daily death tolls. Live-action police brutality caught on cell phone cameras. Rising income inequality, growing food bank lines, and growing house renovation projects. Even more family drama. To mask or not to mask. To vaccinate or not to vaccinate. Not to mention the most ridiculous election in US history.

And seemingly overnight, my clients stopped talking about happiness.

Instead, for a year and a half, all I heard was "I can't wait for things to go back to normal."

4

I think we forgot that normal wasn't really working for us in the first place. My guess is that by the time this book is in your hands, we will have remembered again.

NEW NORMAL OR OLD NORMAL: IT'S ALL RELATIVE

Anyone who lived through 2020 knows that normal is relative. What were once considered clinically significant behaviors became routines of our everyday lives. What do I mean by this? If a patient had told me, at any other point in my career, that she was sanitizing her groceries with disinfecting wipes, wearing a mask every time she went out in public, and washing her hands eight to ten times a day *in addition to* using hand sanitizer? That would have been a no-brainer diagnosis: obsessive-compulsive disorder.

Until it became our normal.

Now that the risk of contracting a global virus is no longer a major threat, I would have to question that behavior once again if someone would present with it in my office. I would assess what motivates my patient to do these things. I would consider what her everyday life looked like—including risk factors like a sick family member—if she was mentally stable, and why she needed such extreme measures to feel safe. And after considering all those factors, I would have to ask the most important question: Is this behavior working for her? Certainly it doesn't take a cognitive psychotherapist to know this once *normal* behavior might no longer be *healthy*.

Yet how many times do I see people engaging in "normal," culturally acceptable activities—things that everyone else is doing—to the detriment of their own physical, mental, and spiritual health? How often do I watch whole families doing what is perfectly "normal": overscheduling themselves and their children, overspending, overposting every detail of their lives? And please know that I am including myself in this category. Therapists are human too. (I need a T-shirt that says that.) In our culture of excess, we all do things that we *know* aren't good for us, that we *know* don't make us happy. But we don't do anything to change because everyone else is doing these things too!

It's normal.

Yet who ever said that normal meant healthy? From the research, we know normal certainly doesn't mean happy.

If we stop assessing our lives and just keep living in this version of "normal," we could miss what is healthy. If we continue wiping down our groceries and obsessively washing our hands when the risk of a virus is gone, this old normal now becomes pathological and mentally unhealthy. When we just accept and settle into what's normal, we stop asking some very important questions that can lead us to the truth of what we truly need in life—questions like "Is this working for me or my family?" Maybe what's right for us doesn't look normal. The very things that look abnormal in our culture may bring us to a level of health that "normal" never will.

THE QUESTION I GET EVERYWHERE

As soon as people find out I'm a therapist, they tell me a story. I can tell by the look of relief in their eyes that it's coming. It doesn't matter where I am: on the soccer field sidelines, in line at the grocery store, at a cocktail party, on a cross-Atlantic flight, at our local bakery, or even on the table of my ob-gyn. I have heard so many personal stories from people who don't even know me—and don't give a fudgesicle who else is listening. Once they find an empathetic ear, they're off and running. I've heard from people I just met about their STD diagnosis, the bizarre thing their teenage son did over the weekend, the possibility that their distracted child has ADD, their husband's patent leather high-heel fetish, or that weird rash they developed overnight. (When did I become a dermatologist?)

Sometimes this gets a tad bit tiring, especially when I just want to quietly grab a chocolate croissant, run out of that bakery, and eat it in my car before I get home so I don't have to share it with my kids. My fourteen-year-old daughter says that this problem is completely my fault because I tell people what I do for work; she suggests that I say I'm an accountant, because "no one wants to talk to an accountant." (I once told that story when we were out for drinks with a couple we were just getting to know, and of course, the husband turned out to be an accountant.)

I listen to these people, though, because I know there is a question underneath their story. I hear the anxiety in their voice. It's easy to identify when you have experienced it yourself. I know that question behind their stories very well. Sometimes they articulate the question; sometimes they don't. Regardless, it is the same one that presents itself in every dilemma I hear: "Is this normal?"

Sure, there are variations: "Am I normal?" "Is he or she normal?" But the urgency that is usually behind the question is hard to dismiss. It is almost like if I answer yes to that question, then they will think everything is going to be OK. But as most of us have experienced, that is often not the case.

Is it normal for teenagers to cut themselves? Is it normal that couples get dissatisfied with their marriages and have affairs? Is it normal for women to get breast cancer in their forties? Is it normal that mass shootings occur each day in the US? If "normal" means things that happen often, then yes. Anxiety is so normal now that we might as well sell Lexapro-infused bottled water (now there's a billion-dollar thought). But these are normals most of us would never want. So why do we settle for normals that we know don't fulfill us? The next few chapters will begin to unpack exactly why.

In short, we have adjusted ourselves to a normal in which kids have no downtime, adults are exhausted working for a life they don't have time to enjoy, and families and relationships suffer due to both. Why do these normals seem so acceptable and even desirable? At some point, we have to pause and consider, Is our collective declining mental health, decreased life satisfaction, and pervasive stress connected to our normal? And what is the cost we are paying to sustain it? From what I have witnessed in more than sixteen years of practice and in my own life, I can tell you: the cost is very, very high.

IS HAPPINESS THE GOAL?

In 2020, I stopped asking my clients what would make them happy. The answers I had received in sessions before 2020 almost didn't seem possible or relevant anymore. *Traveling, finding a new job, getting in shape, spending more time with people I care about*: no one was talking about these things anymore. These ideas about what we thought would make us happy? In light of our new terrifying reality, they actually sounded trivial. While most of us certainly had more time on our hands and thus more opportunity to do some of those things, stress and uncertainty permeated this new situation, which turned life as we knew it upside down. We tested our coping mechanisms, good and bad, to max capacity. The things once in the shadows of our lives—relationship issues, addictions, various -isms, mild mood disorders—didn't just come into the light. It was as if the pandemic held up a powerful magnifying glass to them, and they became blindingly impossible to avoid.

My questions during that time probed deeper. That year our focus became survival, both emotional and physical. Happiness seemed superficial, devoid of depth, and incapable of healing the open wounds caused by months of disconnect, loss, and grief. I found myself constantly asking my clients, "What can you do that calms you?" "What would bring you a moment of peace?" and "What can you still do under these circumstances that would be meaningful to you?"

In the midst of uncertainty, fear, and frustration, these questions forced my clients to do several things. They had to tap into their innermost reserves of strength, accept the situation with all its limitations, stretch their mental bandwidth to think of new possibilities, and step into their power of agency. The results never ceased to amaze me. I began to witness a resilience that I hadn't seen before. I heard people expressing gratitude for things that we took for granted every single day.

And perhaps most significantly, I watched people discover something far more powerful than happiness, something that was not dependent on this incomprehensible situation: contentment.

According to the *Merriam-Webster Collegiate Dictionary*, contentment (as in the state of being contented) is "feeling or showing satisfaction with one's possessions, status, or situation." In other words, to be content is to be satiated by or at peace with what you have, who you are, or the life you are living. In *other* other words, contentment is the feeling of *enough*.

Simply stated, if happiness is defined by having everything you want, contentment is wanting everything you have.

Contentment is the deep appreciation of *enough*. Contentment recognizes that enough is sufficient, satisfying, peaceful yet powerful. Living with an attitude of enough frees us from those things that hold us captive. Enough always sees the beauty of the life we have been given exactly as it is.

Happiness is bold yet fleeting. It's strong in the moment yet often quickly blows into the horizon by the winds of constantly changing emotions, situations beyond our control, and our ever-increasing desire for more of whatever brought it around in the first place. When happiness is present, it's important that we breathe it in deeply and feel the power of its spirit-elevating presence. We can hold on to these moments and remember them when the everyday challenges of life appear, strengthening and lifting us when we need them the most.

Contentment is quieter than happiness, somewhat subtle, yet more powerful than it appears. Its roots run deep and wide so that it stands firm, unchanged by the shifting sands of unexpected situations and overwhelming emotions. We find an unshakeable force within contentment, one that keeps us grounded despite a world that is constantly moving toward bigger, better, and more. Contentment is what keeps us on the path and enables us to see beauty in the uneven ground beneath our feet. Contentment savors the unexpected streams discovered along the way and the crisp chill of the evening air. Most importantly, contentment always recognizes how far we've traveled since we started the journey.

OK, let me break it down for you like this: If you walked into your closet, happiness would be that gorgeous, flowy scarlet-red dress and sparkly stilettos. Or perhaps it's that bold, bright-blue power suit you wore when you had that big presentation in front of the board. Contentment is that well-worn, tattered sweatshirt that you pick 95 percent of the time because you want to feel cozy, warm, and relaxed. At some point, you get tired of the dress and find a new suit, but that sweatshirt? Irreplaceable. Major staying power.

Although I had thought about the topic of contentment well before 2020, during that year, I saw the practices that lead to a content and meaningful existence rise up and come to life. Those clients and friends who practiced them emerged from that trying year stronger, calmer, and more resilient. They came out of quarantines and health scares, job changes and serious family conflicts with hope, stories of incredible gratitude, and even memorable moments. Those who could not access those practices of contentment survived, but they seemed to have lost something of themselves along the way. They were left drained with little motivation, sometimes irreconcilable sadness, and even worse, regret.

And there ended my quest to write a book on happiness. So no, this book won't make you happy. Happiness is no longer what I'm after. I know it will come and go in my life and in yours—*that's* normal. But what if I could help you find contentment? Contentment appears to be something of a super-power, able to withstand even life's most difficult situations while gently leading one down the path of peace, purpose, and meaning. Who wouldn't want that?

THE DISCLAIMER

I don't have some holy grail answer that will instantly transform how you feel and change your life in an instant. The practices that will lead to contentment and fulfillment that we will explore in the second half of this book are just that: practices. Researchers in science, psychology, philosophy, and religion have agreed that these age-old, common postures cultivate a life of calm and fulfillment. I will also show you helpful concepts from several modalities of therapies that I use with clients. These include cognitive behavioral therapy (CBT), mindfulness-based stress reduction (MBSR), dialectical behavioral therapy (DBT), and acceptance commitment therapy (ACT), all of which will help you find your center of calm in most circumstances.

I call these practices the "keys to contentment," which might sound mysterious or even magical, but they are pretty basic and straight up take some work. To be honest with you, initially, they are even boring. You can't wait to get started, right?

But can I tell you something?

They work.

Not just work—they *really work*. As in, they work in a freaking (that's the nice word) global pandemic.

How do I know this? One day during the time of the novel coronavirus, my four kids were at home, learning remotely. I was making lunch like a short-order cook at a greasy diner—on top of seeing patients all day on my iPad, might I add. As I hurried around the kitchen, I noticed my then six-year-old daughter, Carolina, quietly tiptoeing with her Chromebook into our family room. She stood there with a mischievous glint in her eyes and turned her laptop screen toward the television. She had lost interest in her livestream writing class, so she had decided that she'd watch a show instead of practicing her writing . . . *and* that her whole kindergarten class should watch the show too.

My husband and I looked at each other. At this point, we had spent way too much together time during lockdown, learning fun new things about each other like who breathes louder while eating. (It's not me.) "I hope you can see that I really can be content in *any* situation," I told him as I calmly took a deep breath and let the situation be. After all, it *was* a good show.

I even laughed—and maybe cried a little too—but I didn't lose it.

It was because of these practices.

You will learn the neuroscience behind them, which helps us understand why these practices are so effective. And once you commit to them, they become addictive in the best way possible. People, calm is addictive. It is also contagious. So don't be surprised when your friends start to ask you what happened, because, girl, they will want what you ordered! If you are a man, you know most men usually don't talk to one another about this kind of thing, according to my husband, but my guess is your friends will know something is up.

So now you know why I couldn't promise that this book will make you happy. I don't think any book that makes that promise can truly deliver on it. What I *do* promise this book will do for you is give you the questions you need to ask yourself to create a life that is right for you. That is what good therapy does: helps you ask the right questions to discover the answers that are best for *you*. This is not a one-size-fits-all kind of life.

You, your people, and your situations are unique. Take the time and think these choices through. There is too much at stake if you don't.

When you begin to implement the keys, expect stops and starts. This is not an all-or-nothing journey. That kind of process never really works for humans anyway. And if there is one thing you will learn as you begin, it's that we are so very, beautifully human.

A LITTLE ABOUT ME

I want to share a few more things with you before we continue. First, I have always wished I could be the kind of writer who leaves you with those transformative, flowery metaphors that stay with you for the rest of your life. But that's not me—especially these days, when 70 percent of my written correspondences take the form of emojis or GIFs (awesome ones, but still). I think of myself more as a speaker than as a writer. Talking is my comfort zone. I've been talking to people for sixteen years in therapy as an anxiety specialist. On my podcast, *All Things Life*, I love talking with people pretty much about all the things. So I decided that I was going to write this book to you as if you were sitting with me at my kitchen counter over coffee or, let's be honest, a spicy jalapeño margarita. I make really good ones. Sometimes as I wrote this book, I even imagined that I was texting you. (I even tried to put emojis in this book, but my publisher nixed that.) Writing a book literally hurt my brain on some days. But I felt strongly that I needed to write this one and get it into your hands. Stay with me, and I'll tell you that story at the end.

Second, my faith is a big part of my journey and, in addition to psychology, the lens through which I see everything. As a Tamil American, I have family members who are Christian, Hindu, and Buddhist. These are the three most common religions on the island of Sri Lanka, where my parents grew up. Although I am a Christian, I have learned a lot through conversations with family members who were raised in other religious traditions. I believe we can find some of the same life-directing truths resonating in many places. Interestingly enough, the Judeo-Christian tradition substantiates each of the eight practices we examine in the second part of this book. Many of them can also be found in seven of the world's most practiced religions. When you look for truth, you will find it. It is hard to miss when it is spoken of in so many different places.

You may not believe in God, or spirituality may not even be a thought for you, and that's OK. This book can still work for you. I am a Columbia University–trained psychotherapist by trade, and unbiased objectivity is the foundation of my career. After over a decade and a half of private practice, I have been told that my clients feel heard and accepted, and I am hopeful that they leave feeling stronger and more empowered than when they first walked through my office door. I approach this book very much like I approach my clients. In these pages, I will share what I have experienced in my faith when appropriate, and only because it is my lived experience and one that I hope will encourage you. These spiritual moments have inspired me, directed me, and filled me in a way that nothing else in this life has. I have known unusual revelation and peace deep in my mind and soul that are hard to explain in mere words. Do with this information about my life of faith what you will. Receive it deeply, or take it with a grain of salt.

Regardless of your beliefs, the purely psychological principles and methods detailed in this book are rooted in research and stand alone. The efficacy of these treatments has been proven in research-based practice, and I will distill some of that research here. I have also seen these practices work in the lives of hundreds of my patients, and I am confident they will help you too.

As therapists, we are trained not to self-disclose. There is a reason for that. Your process is your process. If your therapist is talking more than you are in therapy—if you know more about her life than your own issues—well, Houston, we have a problem. (Seriously, red-flag those sessions!) Clearly I have already violated that protocol in this book, and we haven't even made it to chapter 2! Yet experts encourage therapists to self-disclose if that can move a person forward in their own process. For that reason, I do share about myself in this book: stories from my life, my perspective on contentment, and strategies that have enabled me to adopt these practices.

I did not want this book to overwhelm you with information or become another to-do list. At the end of each chapter in part II, there are a few simple steps to help you "turn the key" and get started with each practice. I suggest you focus on one, put the book down, practice, implement, and when you are ready for more, pick it up again.

Having said that, the questions I ask throughout the book are just as important as the methods. Spend some time thinking through those questions. You can even imagine me sitting across from you in my therapy chair, staring at you silently for an awkwardly long time, awaiting your response. Yup, that's pretty much therapy in a nutshell. But it's amazing the answers that emerge out of that silence—after all, the silence is where we begin to find our inner voice of wisdom. In this space, my clients often find the answers to the very questions they are asking.

My hope is that you will find a few practices that you connect with and that bring you a bit of daily calm in this hectic pace of life we all maintain. If you walk away from this book implementing just one change or finding a new idea that brings you a little more clarity or experiencing just a bit more peace—well, I consider that a win for both of us.

But first, if we are talking about contentment and how to find it, we have to begin with examining the pervasive influences in our culture that prevent us from experiencing it.

If you are anything like me, what you are about to discover will astound you—not only because truth, when uncovered, can be shocking but more likely because some of this truth hits far too close to home. I can't be the only one who looks at life as we know it and thinks, *This is completely . . . crazy!*

CHAPTER 2

Crazy

If Crazy Town had a mayor, I would be unanimously elected. I constantly find myself down the hall in my colleague Lisa's office, asking, "Can you figure out what's wrong with me?" Lisa is a psychologist and one of my closest friends. We've run a therapy practice together for more than twelve years. "Just ten minutes on your couch," I plead. "You're so good. I know you can do it."

True confessions from your therapist. Encouraging, right? *I'm* the one telling you how to find calm and contentment? But the struggle is real for all of us, and I know it all too well. Even therapists get swept up in the tides of madness disguised as normalcy.

I show Lisa a photo of the color-coded spreadsheet of my kids' spring schedule. I have four children, each with their own world of scholastic commitments and extracurricular activities. I swipe to my iCal, which is also color coded for each child and shared with my five other family members so we all know what's up with one another. Activities change every season, and so does my driving schedule. I've got it down to a pink, purple, green, and blue science. Soccer, swim, lacrosse, ballet, guitar:

the list goes on, and of course no one is on the same field at the same time. Generally speaking, children of Puerto Ricans and Sri Lankans—Puerto-Lankans, if you will—aren't known for their athletic prowess. I mean, I'm pretty certain my kids will not be Olympic athletes. So why are they training like them at nine years old?

Can you see why I am ecstatic when someone wants to quit something? I practically anoint that kid with oil as I give my most sincere blessing to be a quitter. Some days I spend several hours in the car and drive close to fifty miles for their extracurriculars—all without even leaving town. I *know* this is nuts. But I have been doing it for more than a decade, because here in my sweet town, kids start achieving before they can walk. And God forbid you as a parent don't give them the same opportunities that their friends have.

Actually, I sometimes stop and ask myself, What *would* happen if my kids didn't have the same opportunities their friends have? What if we jumped off the hamster wheel of "Well, everyone does it"? *Then* what?

Most of us—myself included—get a sinking feeling in our stomachs when we briefly consider that option. And we don't think much further than that. Thought dismissed. Because *crazy* is the not-so-new normal—and I'm a therapist, so you know I don't throw around that c-word lightly. And yes, I rearrange everything—my life, my patient schedule, our family time (or lack thereof)—all of it to accommodate it. To accommodate crazy.

But why do I do this? As a clinician, I see the impact of this type of keeping-up culture on our collective mental and physical health. I know better. The answer is so simple and yet so complex at the same time: pressure.

THE HUSTLE

If someone would ask me, "Do you feel pressure to do what everyone else does?" my immediate response would be a resounding no! I'm not one to cave to other people's expectations, and I've always thought of myself as an independent thinker. Both of these qualities were reinforced when I attended a women's college, which gave me a new lens on the importance of thinking for myself not just as a woman but as a person of color. And while I'm only five-feet-nothing on a good day and can barely see over the steering wheel of my SUV, I'm the one everyone in my family calls to deal with people who are acting obnoxious. "Talk to them; they will listen to you," my sisters tell me. "You're tiny but tough," my mom always says. Lisa even calls me "the heavy" in our business partnership, as I'm usually the one to deal with conflict-related issues.

Yet pressure comes in many forms. Even when it is subtle and covert, it can still powerfully influence our choices and shape our own self-perception and even self-worth.

Pressure often travels with its ride or die: expectation. In our achievement- and success-oriented culture, we are expected to do a lot and to do it well. We earn our worthiness around here, thank you very much! Expectations are often unspoken, but we are more than aware of them. These are the unwritten rules that, if followed, promise great rewards. Whether you are a stay-at-home or employed parent, a single woman, or a married man, you face cultural and societal expectations that, when met, increase your sense of accomplishment, desirability, social influence, and value. All these things do impact our self-worth and—dare I even suggest—our *happiness*.

In today's world, there's pressure to be a good wife and mother. You've got to raise those kids well—meaning well rounded and involved in everything—so they have a shot at a decent college. Sure, you're an educated woman, so you have your career, but maybe you need to start your own business or find a side hustle, because one job is clearly not enough—and besides, everyone's got a side hustle. You always manage to fit in your regular barre or Pilates or—better yet—Peloton workouts. Sure, those might have to be at 5:45 a.m., but you gotta do what you gotta do. You know your *why*, right? Your word for the year? Your mantra?

Oh, and put healthy, gluten-free, dairy-free, taste-free meals that your kids will eat on the table every night. In your free time, go out to coffee with your friends and women you don't know—or really like, for that matter—because mom friendships can make or break your kids' social life. Volunteer at your kids' school, especially on class party days, even if you have to call in sick to make it happen. Heck, be the class mom, because otherwise, your kids will complain that you are never there. Always return texts and emails and DMs from your four social media platforms promptly or else people will think you don't care and you will lose followers. Post about snow days—which always means sledding, hot chocolate, and freshly baked snowflake cookies. Spend forever looking for the photo where it looks like the kids actually did the decorating (forget that they were in the kitchen only five minutes before your daughter kicked your son for touching her arm accidentally). From 4 to 8 p.m., drive back and forth to various activities—and, oh yes, don't forget to reserve that last bit of gas in the tank when you hit the bedroom at 11 p.m. Your partner is waiting eagerly because it's been days . . .

This is the hustle.

Does any one person have the patience, stamina, and ability to do it all?

We have been led to believe the more you hustle, the stronger, smarter, and more accomplished you are. We have to earn our worthiness, right? But don't forget—the more you hustle, the more exhausted, disconnected, and distracted you are too.

Men feel the weight of the hustle as well as women. I've witnessed that struggle in my clients and even in my own husband: working in a culture where enough is never enough—and that means long days, long commutes, playing the game to get ahead. What do you do? What car do you drive? What zip code do you live in? Get to the gym, be strong. Emotions? Be vulnerable, but don't feel too much—we don't want *that*. Be a great partner, and with that extra time you have, show up at every school play, coach the basketball team, and be a great father too.

It's all too much.

Do you think anyone is really crushing it? Or is *it* crushing *us*?

Think for a moment beyond social media. Therapists are often privy to the backstory that you never see on Instagram or Facebook. I've given you a glimpse into mine at the start of this book. Not what you'd expect from a therapist, right? You might be surprised that people you think have it together in every area of their lives still have their stuff. Trust me, some of that stuff runs deep. Those picture-perfect social media feeds? Therapist protip: they often belong to people who are struggling the most.

This pace is unrealistic for any human.

And because we are human, we make mistakes, we fall short, and we can't meet these unrealistic expectations for ourselves on our *best* day, let alone our worst. We all drop the ball at some point trying to keep up the hustle. Hear me on this: we all are *not* enough sometimes.

Feeling not enough is part of the reason that we live with insecurity, and insecurity craves validation. We look for ways to affirm that we are OK, normal, and, most important, worthy. So we keep trying, no matter the cost to our own or our family's mental and physical health.

So I like to imagine that I am making my own choices and thinking for myself. But occasionally, I stop and take a closer look at these moments, and I ask myself, "Why are we doing this?" Answers to *why* questions are often hard to find. We don't always know *why* we do the things we do; we just know *that* we do them. Perhaps a better question—one that I love to use in therapy sessions—is "What is making me do this?"

I ask myself this every time we go skiing.

THE PRESSURE COOKER

My husband and I are island people, just one generation removed: his family from Puerto Rico, mine from Sri Lanka. To us, there's no better vacation than eighty-degree sun, sand, and sea. We didn't grow up skiing. In fact, our parents would *never* have considered paying a small fortune to throw themselves down a snow-covered mountain. There's a reason you can't spot many brown folks on ski mountains—they aren't there.

"Why stay out in the cold for hours, risking your life, when you can be inside in the heat?" Even now, as we stuff six pairs of cold-weather everything into an already packed SUV, I can practically hear the disapproval in my mother's voice, her Sri Lankan accent still strong after almost fifty years in America. There are certain things my immigrant parents will never find entertaining. Skiing is one, and camping is the other. The idea of people actually wanting to sleep outside on the ground in a place with no bathrooms—for *fun*—is beyond these two. They came to America so we would never have to do that.

Yet here we are, doing the things that make no sense to our parents. Honestly, I agree with them on camping. I activate the house alarm every night, so why would we sleep outside nicely wrapped in a sleeping-bag bow for serial killers *and* bears? But something within me thinks my kids should know how to ski. It is good for their mental health in the winter, gets them off their devices, and gives them time outside when the weather in Connecticut is less than inviting. But I recognize another motivation, subtle but just as compelling. So many other kids go skiing, and I don't want my children to feel left out, now or later on, when their friends want to do this together. I want them to have the option, even as I'm f-bombing all the way down the mountain. (I really, *really* try not to.) Could you say skiing makes them more desirable or increases their social capital? Perhaps. Whatever it is, it's strong enough to overcome my chocolate-covered, island-loving genetics.

If I am truly making my own choices based solely on what I think is best for me and my family, I've got a lot of questions for myself. Why am I always trying the latest weight loss fitness challenge, even when I know I'm at a healthy weight? Why do I want a pair of shoes that I didn't really like at first but saw so many times on other people that they grew on me? Why do I care to suddenly visit certain places that I felt absolutely fine not visiting because apparently everyone has been there?

You might be thinking by now that I'm talking about pressures and expectations unique to middle- and upper-middle-class suburbanites. It's true that pressures and expectations take specific forms in specific locations. But having worked as a social worker in economically distressed Brooklyn neighborhoods and now running a private practice in privileged Fairfield County, Connecticut, I can say this: comparison and competition are part of our human nature and our natural evolution. Regardless of our socioeconomic status, we struggle with this. Our brains are actually wired to take in information, make comparisons, and determine the right thing to do, think, or say. Comparison serves as a *heuristic*, or mental shortcut, that helps us make good decisions quickly. Yes, comparing can be beneficial, yet clearly in this context of achievement and worthiness, it is no longer helpful.

What we are dealing with here is pressure to do more, be more, and have more. Internalizing the expectation that we should do it all (which, remember, was never realistic in the first place), we feel insecure, stressed, and anxious when we can't. We then search for validation that we are still OK, accepted, and worthy . . . which loops us back to the beginning of this cycle. Maybe if I can do more, be more, be seen more, or have more—maybe then I will feel good about myself . . . and be happy.

SEARCHING FOR PURPOSE

Our culture these days seems to pressure us to find our purpose, fight for happiness, and unleash our passions. We deserve *more* than life is offering us right now. The message "You are made for *more*" floods our feeds. But what if we don't know what our passion is? What if we haven't defined our purpose? Then the *more* we search for only leads to more insecurity, more uncertainty, and more frustration.

Many of my clients experience great stress when it comes to finding purpose, so it's a topic that frequently comes up in sessions. Earlier I described the pressure I feel to get everything done for everyone. We often feel pressure to do what we feel called to do. We see others living their lives well, succeeding, crushing it. But life as we know it—real life—is full of challenges, so it may not feel like we are at the same level. The images we see and stories we hear that shape our perception of others make us question our own worth. What are we contributing to our families? What are we contributing to the world? The idea of purpose even takes on an air of altruism, which makes it easily palatable and seemingly essential. Fulfilling one's purpose then can become an almost tangible measure of our value as humans. This is where it becomes dangerous. We don't need to earn our value as human beings. Adults can agree that children are worthy of love and are inherently valuable simply because they are children. We need to affirm that adults are inherently valuable too.

Yet many of us don't see it this way, and our culture does not reinforce such a message. Instead, we feel pressure. We all know what happens when pressure builds and has nowhere to go. For this reason, we are seeing astronomically high rates of burnout: emotional, mental, and physical exhaustion caused by unrelenting stress.

Exhaustion affects every area of our lives. Plain and simple: many of us are too tired to be happy.

And this continuous striving for what we think will ultimately bring happiness?

How's that working out for us?

FIRST WORLD PROBLEMS: THE DECLINE OF HAPPINESS

According to the World Happiness Report (WHR), a survey that polls 156 countries, the world's state of happiness doesn't look promising. The WHR asks, "Taken all together, how would you say things are these days—would you say that you are very happy, pretty happy or not too happy?"

The WHR, in addition to other polls on happiness, clearly depicts our reality in the United States, and similar findings in the United Kingdom and Australia suggest a parallel trend:

- Since 2012, happiness in the United States has been on the decline.

- In 2019, before the global pandemic, the United States reported an all-time low in life satisfaction.

- According to the same study, which was confirmed in Gallup research, the United States dropped to number nineteen in the world for reported happiness. This is one spot lower than in 2018 and five spots below its 2017 ranking.

- In 2020, according to an NBC poll, only 14 percent of US adults reported that they were happy. Although this poll was taken during the coronavirus pandemic, according to the data collected and studied since 1972 by the General Social Survey, we were clearly headed in that direction even without a global pandemic.

This is not OK. What is going on? Who is really winning here?

Many of us feel trapped in this never-ending hustle for happiness. This toxic cycle takes a serious toll on our mental and physical health. In order to find true contentment, we have to break this cycle. It's no wonder that we are looking at the greatest mental health issues our world has ever seen and that those numbers continue to increase annually.

And here's a sobering truth: it's not just affecting us as adults. We are now passing it down from generation to generation.

WHAT HAPPENED TO A HAPPY CHILDHOOD?

According to the same World Happiness Report, adolescents—a demographic that experienced a rise in life satisfaction and happiness from 1991 to 2011—experienced a sudden decline from 2012 to the present. Each year the report on adolescent well-being is worse than the one before.

Interestingly enough, social media platforms such as Facebook and Instagram exploded in revenue and popularity in 2012. We observed a direct correlation to the decline of adolescent mental health at the very same time. Social media plays a large role in what we are seeing, both statistically and in practice, and we will look at this correlation more in the following chapters.

Any working therapist can anecdotally affirm this is true. In 2019, it proved a challenge to find an adolescent therapist who had availability in their schedule and was taking new clients.

By 2021, it was nearly impossible. Along with the decline in happiness, we saw an increase in depression and in suicidal ideation and self-harm, especially for girls and young women. The suicide rate is growing exponentially for kids aged seven to ten. That's as young as first grade, people. These statistics also proved true across the pond, for children and youth in the United Kingdom.

If you're a parent or caregiver, take just a minute to think about the kids you are raising; if you don't have kids, think about the kids you know. Do their lives look anything like yours did when you were growing up? Do you remember what you were doing in the first grade? I'm pretty sure it wasn't spending three or four hours on a screen. It doesn't matter if you are twenty or seventy-five: there has been a marked change in the last several years, and it isn't a good one. Colleges are recruiting kids earlier, sending information about their programs to students as young as the seventh grade. Kids in elementary schools have very little unstructured play or free time, which is vital for their social and emotional development. Playdates are scheduled and often supervised by a parent—one who has taken it upon themselves to structure the "unstructured time" with elaborate projects—such as, for example, creating Venetian glass-beaded potholders. I exaggerate, but not by much. (And an FYI: I set up playdates for my kids so I don't have to play with them, so do you think I'm about to play with yours?)

Seasonal sports are now practiced year-round, so kids who once played multiple sports have to choose only one—and this starts as early as the third grade. Many kids who do choose to play two sports per season experience the problem of overscheduling, as practices are often held several times a week. I know parents who spend three hours in their car several times a week driving their ten-year-olds to Russian math lessons. I know parents whose eight-year-olds attend outdoor soccer clinics in twenty-degree weather to get them ready for the travel team four years in advance. I know parents who have their fourteen-year-olds take SAT practice tests once a month to prepare them three years in advance for the real deal. As you can see, we have created a world where our kids are hustling too.

Much like a highly transmissible virus, our need for validation through achievement now replicates itself in our kids. And many of us appease our own insecurities, our own unresolved need for validation, through the success of our children.

I will never forget when my then thirteen-year-old daughter, Natalia, schooled her therapist mama on the importance of balance. (This is the daughter who told me I should tell people I'm an accountant—I know, smart kid.)

That year, she had to decide if she was going to join a popular volunteer organization in our town. Volunteering sounds great, right? But many girls join this organization essentially to check off the "I'm a good person" box for college applications. I had received a text from a mother I didn't really know offering to be Natalia's sponsor so she could join (apparently you need one of those).

My friends and I were talking about whether adding yet another commitment to our kids' overscheduled lives was a good thing. The response I consistently received was "Well, you know colleges love it." A few friends whose daughters were years deep into this organization, however, vehemently discouraged me from doing it. "Seriously, you need this like you need another baby," one told me. Oh, *hell* no; that was all I needed to hear. (We all need friends who can speak our language and give us perspective when we've lost it. Hold on to them: they are your people.)

I asked Natalia what she thought and if she wanted to join. She thought about it and said a firm no. "If people really don't care about volunteering, then I don't see the point of joining," she said simply. "I am swimming five days a week, focusing on school, and I want some free time to spend with my friends. Some downtime. Maybe we can do some volunteer work as a family like we did on Thanksgiving."

I didn't accept this answer at first. I challenged, "Are you sure? Many of your friends are doing it. You kind of have to decide now. I don't want you to regret it." Nice one, anxiety-specialist mom. (This is where I really need the smack-my-head brown girl emoji. I really miss emojis. So much you can say in one little face.)

But she didn't flinch. "I'm sure."

And she was right. This kid has always had a calm confidence that surprises me. She made her choices, avoided drama, and was not easily swayed by what everyone else was doing. She grew up having a new sibling every couple of years since she was two years old. I credit her strong sense of autonomy to my preoccupation with the busyness of younger kids. (That's certainly better than living in the mom-guilt of worrying that she was neglected; talk about convenient reframing.) It's amazing what happens when we step back and let our kids figure things out themselves. And when you take that step back, pay attention: the kids often become *our* teachers.

Meanwhile, Charity Tiger Mom was texting me regularly, asking if we had made a decision about joining the organization—I mean, like almost every day. I was starting to wonder if she got a kickback from our membership. I politely told her that Natalia was committed to swimming and her schoolwork and did not want to take it on right now. That should be enough, right?

This well-meaning, surprisingly persistent woman I hardly knew countered my nonoffer. For real. "Oh, well so many of the girls in her middle school class who swim are doing it," she texted. "And BTW—it would look great on her college application."

And with that, she threw the gasoline on my Sri Lankan American fire. Was she implying that my kid was *less than* because she didn't want another commitment? Didn't this woman know not to mess with a brown mama's babies? And why did I even care? As I said, I didn't even know this woman! Why couldn't I just calmly take this in stride and say, "Thanks, but we're good!"

Yet deep down, I knew my reaction had nothing to do with this woman. I was not reacting to her; I was reacting to my feelings about pressure. This is exactly the type of pressure that I see in the office: expectations that force kids to take on too much. And then we're surprised that they suffer from debilitating anxiety when they cannot meet the demands of their choices (or ours). And who is left to "fix it" and answer parents' questions, like "How many sessions do you think this will take?"

So I was angry—both on behalf of my own daughter (who couldn't care less, by the way) and on behalf of my stressed-out, anxious teenaged clients. I don't remember what I texted back, but I'm sure it was strong. Whatever I wrote, I figured it was better than the middle-finger emoji. Like any calm, mature professional, however, I did take to social media to air my grievance and posted this:

Dear Parents,

Please respect other parents' decision to NOT talk to their seventh grader about what looks good on their college application. OK? Thanks!

Love,
Your Local Therapist Trying to Prevent
High Schoolers from Stress-Induced
Panic Attacks in Ninth Grade

This post ended up garnering quite a bit of attention, including a repost from a *New York Times* bestselling author of "How to Raise an Adult," Julie Lythcott-Haims. Many parents in our community wholeheartedly agreed, aware of the epidemic of adolescent anxiety. Even the mom who inspired my post commented, "Absolutely!"—self-awareness clearly not a strong point.

But I get it. At the end of the day, I'm sure that that woman had good intentions. And while I was annoyed at her approach, I'm sure I have my own ridiculous expectations that must make my own kids feel the exact same way.

As parents, we have to do better than this. If we haven't found our own happiness in striving for attainment, why do we keep doing it and reinforcing it in our children? Have you seen that definition of insanity that says it's doing the same things over and over again and expecting a different result? I cannot think of a better description for what we are seeing, year after year. Trying harder to meet the demands of these terms will not bring us any closer to contentment. Pair this with the rates of anxiety, depression, and suicide increasing exponentially at younger and younger ages. We are not getting any happier. Clearly we are not getting healthier either.

The consequences of doing things the same way are too high now. When one out of four college students is contemplating suicide, change is no longer an option; it is an emergency. We owe it to our youth, and we owe it to ourselves.

As you know if you have ever been in therapy: change is not easy, but it is *always* possible. We can't always change our situation, but we can *always* change how we perceive it and how we respond to it. This choice is at the core of finding true contentment. The process might be unfamiliar and even uncomfortable at first, as we will learn when we get into part II. I do believe, though, if we are open to seeing things in a new light, we will find a healthier way to satisfy our truest desires.

Keep in mind that I usually get pushback or resistance from clients when the process gets boring or tough or the solution is incredibly underwhelming. My response? "That's fine," I say. "You can keep doing it the way you want. But how is that working out for you?"

I think we can agree that it isn't.

Even if this hustle culture remains somewhat out of our control, finding peace and calm in the midst of it is possible. Few of us have the option of escaping our lives for months on end to find meaning. You don't need a monastery in Nepal, a costly yoga retreat, or weeks in meditative silence. Although those places and experiences are of great value, they are just not in the cards for most of us.

The good news is contentment is closer than you think. Yes, it will require awareness, intention, and persistence. But as I tell my clients, change does not have to be drastic to be effective. Given the pressure and the hustle, finding contentment might feel like a battle, but I assure you: this is one worth fighting for.

We need to recognize that this desire to be more, do more, and have more is unquenchable. It's as if we are drinking from a waterfall yet constantly feeling . . . thirsty.

CHAPTER 3

Cravings

It was a gorgeous afternoon in late spring, and I was at the beach for a weekend with a friend I hadn't seen in a while. Life had gotten superbusy for both of us, and we needed a break. As much as I adore my family, twenty-four hours without them is like one long, slow, much-needed exhale.

It was the golden hour, my favorite time of day—when everything in the world turns a warm shade of beautiful. With our toes in the sand, our brown skin warmed by the setting sun, and glasses of chilled rosé in hand—well, this was as close to perfection as I could have hoped for at the end of a long work week. As I took a deep breath of the salty seaside breeze, my friend turned to me, looked up from her phone, and asked, "Have you decided what you are going to do this summer?"

I sighed. "I don't even know what I'm going to do *tomorrow*," I replied.

This was absolutely the truth. It's how I roll most of the time, especially when I'm asked that question in April. I know many moms have their daily summer schedule graphed out, kids all signed up for camps and bags packed before the snow even melts in Connecticut. I'm not one of those.

"I'm trying not to think about it. It stresses me out. I just want to enjoy this." I spread my arms out to embrace all the warmth, sea, and sky and hold on to them just a few minutes longer. It felt almost magical.

"I think that's my problem," she admitted. "It stresses me out *not* to plan ahead. I feel like everything will get booked up, and then we are going to miss our chance. We will miss something amazing."

But she *was* missing something amazing. And I told her so in my gentle, smackdown kind of way.

"You know, I do this all the time," she said. "I'm always on to the next thing while I'm still doing the current thing. And it makes my husband crazy." She got a faraway look in her eyes as she began to connect a few dots between her past and her present. As a therapist, I know that look well, and it's one of my all-time favorites.

She went on: "We took an anniversary trip to Barbados last winter. As we were waiting for our bags at the airport, I started looking on my phone at hotels for another trip I wanted to do in the spring."

"You mean after the trip was over?" I asked. "Like, you had such a great time and couldn't wait for the next trip?"

"No." She shook her head slowly. "We had just arrived. *Before* we even got to the hotel. We hadn't even started that vacation, but I already was onto the next one!"

I paused for effect as I took off my sunglasses and raised my eyebrows. "Girl, you got problems!" I told her after a moment. "We gotta work on this."

BUT WHAT ARE WE *REALLY* MISSING?

My friends get the unfiltered-me therapist. Some things I just can't say to my clients, even though I really, *really* want to. This is one of the reasons therapists don't see friends as clients: we are too emotionally involved. Hopefully they know one of those emotions is love.

What my friend was describing is all too common. As we talked, she described the pressure she felt to create amazing family memories for her kids before they went off to college. She wanted them to have experiences that she did not get to have with her own family. She didn't want them to miss out.

A young client first introduced me to the term *FOMO*—fear of missing out—several years ago. Hearing the ping of a Snapchat notification, she checked her phone and found out that at that very moment, several of her good friends were hanging out together at someone's pool. She had not been invited to this gathering, yet she was on the group message thread and saw the photos. This created *a lot* of distress. "I can't believe they did this to me," she said between gasping breaths.

Although FOMO is not officially listed in the *Diagnostic and Statistical Manual of Mental Disorders*, clinicians know it is a very real thing and that it does not discriminate across generations. FOMO now even has its own entry in *Merriam-Webster*: "fear of not being included in something (such as an interesting or enjoyable activity) that others are experiencing."

What we see on Instagram, Facebook, Snapchat, and the like can serve as the catalyst for this anxious feeling. People with this anxiety have the same symptoms as other anxieties, including negative perseverating thoughts that the person just can't shake, worst-case-scenario thinking, and an inability to sleep. I've watched patients experience physical symptoms as they talk through these situations: excessive tears, increased heart rate, nausea, dizziness, and sudden changes in body temperature.

FOMO is real, and it has very real implications and consequences for the way we choose to live our lives. Although it is described as a fear, FOMO triggers a longing or craving for something that, in that moment, we can't have. Think of waiting behind a velvet rope at a club as the bouncer scans his list but can't find your name. Because we can't have it, we often want it more.

Exclusion and the emotions that go along with it are powerful. Clients tell me about going to events and parties they don't want to attend instead of spending time with the people most important to them. Every week I see adolescents who run with crowds that they know are destructive to their mental, emotional, and physical health instead of finding friends who appreciate them for who they truly are. I see people under incredible financial strain and stress trying to maintain a lifestyle comparable to that of friends who "have it all." We spend our most valuable commodity—time—doing these things we think will satisfy us. Yet as a result, we find ourselves anxious and discontent and wondering why we feel that way.

THE POWER SOURCE OF FOMO

As therapists, we see FOMO and similar emotions not as *the* problem but rather as symptoms of the real problem—the underlying issue that keeps getting us into problematic situations. This is why when I see in therapy a couple who are smoking mad at each other and determined to tell me every single detail of their last fight—well, I'm not all that interested. (Although I pretty much do exactly the same thing when we pay our semiannual visits to our couples' therapist. I need another therapist to tell me I'm wrong because I can't always hear it from my husband. But that's a story for another time.) I need to get underneath the current fight about who left their underwear on the floor for the seventy-fifth time to find the systemic issue that is manifesting in all these "stupid little fights," as I call them in my house. Essentially, I need to find the power source that fuels these fights.

So to truly understand FOMO, we need to get to its source, which has to do with three basic emotional needs:

1. *The need for validation.* We all deal with insecurity about something. Some of these insecurities have deep roots in what we experienced growing up when it came to validation, either the lack thereof or too much. Some insecurities are new and occur as we transition into a new role or experience—something that we may not be familiar with and are in the process of figuring out. Some may be trauma related. You may find yourself asking, "Am I good enough as a partner, parent, worker, or friend?" Or "Am I doing enough to earn my worth and value in this role?"

   Pay attention to those deep-rooted insecurities. If you frequently act out of this need for validation—if self-esteem and confidence have been an issue most of your life, if you've felt anxious and insecure for as long as you can remember—take the steps to address this and work on it. Read books or, better yet, talk to someone who can help. Otherwise, those insecurities will frequently emerge like weeds, tangling and strangling experiences that could be enjoyable but end up being stressful and frustrating. Your need for validation can cause you to make choices that lead to more stress—for both you and those around you.

2. *The need for belonging.* We all need to feel loved and accepted. We need people who get us and people we can relate to. We search for that sense of belonging in different ways throughout different stages. We might feel belonging at one stage of life, but stages end. Kids grow up, friendships change, we move, jobs end, we retire and start over. All these changes impact the evolution of our identity—how we see ourselves, how we think others see us, and how we experience our surroundings. At different points in our lives, we might find we are searching for that place of belonging again.

When we see people coming together and we are on the outside, our sense of belonging feels threatened. We may feel like we are losing our position or place or connection to that group.

3. *The need for pleasure.* Happiness is fleeting and temporary, and as we're learning in this book, contentment is deeper and more sustainable. But happiness *is* pleasurable, so we constantly seek ways to experience it. When we are happy, we feel good, and often the feeling of pleasure is our indication that we are enjoying life. Who doesn't want that?

According to Freud's pleasure principle, we have an instinctive drive to seek pleasure to satisfy both our biological and psychological cravings. Whether or not you are a fan of Freud, it's clear that when we see other people doing things that bring them pleasure, we process that experience as beneficial. In addition, the need for validation and the need to belong also motivate us to experience what others are experiencing.

Problems emerge, however, with *how* we tend to look to fulfill these human needs. We are a culture of instant gratification and quick fixes. Have you ever been appalled to find out the item you ordered online won't get to you for seven to ten business days? (Of course you have—thank you, Amazon Prime.) We do the same thing with other areas of our lives, looking for two-day fixes to meet our needs. So when everyone else is doing something that *seems* to make them happy, we are compelled to do it too.

But when we do, it's like putting a Band-Aid on a gushing, open wound. It holds for a moment, and we feel a bit better. But eventually we need a real solution—one that has some permanence—to stop the bleeding and start the healing.

I want to explain a few things that make us constantly search for happiness rather than find contentment in our lives. Contentment, for one, is countercultural and goes against every marketing strategy that we are bombarded with every time we click a button. What might surprise you is that we are also neurobiologically wired to seek more. Our cravings are due, in part, to a tiny but powerful neurochemical called dopamine.

THAT'S DOPE

There are many ways to make sense of human behavior. History, philosophy, religion, and psychology all offer explanations of why we do the things we do. Although I am a cognitive therapist, I have always been intrigued by the field of neuroscience. It was actually my first major in college—until I realized that neuroscience majors spent most of their days hanging out with rats, and, well, that was not happening.

But the fact that our motivations, actions, and moods are related to tiny molecules circulating in our bodies and produced in response to our changing circumstances? That still fascinates me. Understanding processes at that level brings new insight into behaviors many people aren't aware of. Once my clients understand more about what's going on in their brains, they experience many *aha* moments, which then help them actually change their behavior. For that reason—and the fact that I have always been a science dork—a lot of this book will draw on ideas that emerge from neuroscience.

We often talk about a "dopamine hit" or a "dopamine rush" when we experience something pleasurable: falling in love, buying something, getting a sweet text from a friend. You also hear about dopamine when we talk about addictive behavior, like playing video games or using drugs. In my line of work, we talk about dopamine as one neurochemical of the happiness trifecta: dopamine, serotonin, and oxytocin. Those neurochemicals are released when we do things that cause us to feel good.

Until recently, I had understood dopamine as the chemical that recognizes something pleasurable and then tells our brain,

"Do that again." But this is not entirely the case. Understanding what activates dopamine can give us a window into why we constantly search for something that doesn't quite satisfy—and keep going back for more.

In their book *The Molecule of More*, authors Daniel Lieberman and Michael Long detail that dopamine is related specifically to *new* pleasure. It's the novelty or newness of a certain experience that triggers this exciting, addictive feeling. And guess what? Once that experience is no longer new, we don't see dopamine released any longer. It dissipates. This is why Lieberman and Long call dopamine "the molecule of more." Once pleasurable experiences become ordinary or routine, dopamine is no longer triggered, and so we are compelled to search for more. We look for a *new* way to find the same intensity of pleasure and feel satisfied.

This explains that relationship you had with a partner that at first was passionate but faded over time. It's the reason you might *love* pizza but can't eat it every day (unless you are my son). By day five, you get tired of pizza and crave something different. It also explains what I saw firsthand during a recent holiday season. Within hours of opening their Christmas gifts, my two younger girls were searching for the gift cards that their abuela had mailed to them and were begging us to go to Target right then and there. I know it's not their fault, but that doesn't stop me from saying, "What's wrong with you people? You just got a ton of gifts. Can't you just enjoy them?" After such conversations, I always go on a rant about spoiled kids who have *way* too much stuff—to which my twelve-year-old son, Samuel, usually says something like, "I wonder what evil witch appears in the middle of the night and spoils us rotten." That's when I remind my husband that his sarcasm gene has indeed survived the fittest and will continue to strengthen the next generation.

But this cycle—the constant craving for more—is not just about our overprivileged kids. We do the same in our own adult way. This past holiday season, my husband asked me what I wanted for Christmas. For years, I used to say, "Oh, nothing" (code for "Don't even think about doing nothing, and don't you know me well enough by now that you shouldn't have to ask?"). But this year, when he asked, I mentioned that I really liked a belt I had seen. It wasn't something that I would buy for myself, because I honestly don't think a belt is worth that price tag, but I had seen several people wear it and loved how it looked. On Christmas morning, I opened a beautiful moss-green-and-gold box under the Christmas tree, and there within it was the belt. I took it out of the box and ran my finger over the cool, antique gold metal and soft, smooth leather. I started to think about what event I could wear it to and with which outfit it would look best. If you had asked me in that moment how that new belt made me feel, I probably would have said *happy*.

A few moments later, I placed the belt carefully back in the box, gathered a few gifts in my arms, and made my way to the corner of the living room. There I stacked them in a small pile . . . where I then left that belt for two whole months.

The belt that I had coveted for so long? I completely forgot about it.

This is exactly what happens, people. It's dope. Dopamine, that is—or, rather, the lack thereof. The *anticipation* of pleasure, or a gift, or an event triggers the release of dopamine, which elevates our mood and makes us feel excited. But once we are used to whatever that new thing is? The pleasure fades. The novelty is gone. Once I had received this belt that I had so admired—once it was mine—there was no anticipation. I felt no more excitement or novelty, even though I hadn't even worn it yet!

Neuroscience research gives evidence for this emotional shift. When participants are offered new and pleasurable experiences, we witness surges of dopamine. But once the subject has been exposed repeatedly to the same situation, no matter how pleasure inducing, the dopamine diminishes.

So what do we do? We are neurobiologically wired to seek that type of pleasure again. Yet we don't realize that most of the excitement and happiness come from the *anticipation* of the new thing, *not the actual thing itself.* We look for the next new thing that can trigger that same feeling. But once we have the thing, we don't really notice it or appreciate it like we did at first. Over time, the levels of dopamine wear off, and so does the intensity of pleasure.

Wanting only begets more wanting. When the excitement of anticipation gives way to the ordinary, we begin looking for the next best thing. We begin trying to fulfill this ever-present void created by . . . normalcy.

This cycle can also be explained by the *hedonic treadmill.* *Hedonism* is the pursuit of pleasure. The hedonic treadmill describes the fact that each human being has a "set point," or baseline, of happiness in their lives. After something excites us or triggers a surge of pleasure, we will eventually return to our baseline normal level of happiness. That's called hedonic adaptation. Essentially, pleasurable feelings don't last, but because we experienced pleasure once, we will seek it again. Then eventually we return to the same normal, consistent state . . . and so on. This is the hedonic treadmill, and it just confirms to me that I don't like any sort of treadmill.

What we know about neuroplasticity, or brain adaptation, however, suggests that we can actually increase our normal set point. This is especially great news if you have been someone who has struggled with depression since adolescence or someone whose baseline happiness set point is naturally low. Engaging in the practices that foster contentment, found in part II of this book, will help your neural pathways change and adapt. By doing the work, we can actually rewire our brains to become more positive, peaceful, and content. We can *increase* that baseline happy set point to which we return.

Perhaps you can see how the fear of missing out could stimulate our dopamine circuits, promising a new experience and also triggering our deep desire for belonging and validation. Yet much like an addict who can't satisfy a craving, we might realize we can't be a part of whatever it is we are missing and may be left with frustration, anxiety, and even deep sadness. FOMO is not just some cute acronym to describe what teenagers face in a social media world; it's way more serious than it may sound. I have seen persistent FOMO as a trigger for depression and even suicidal ideation.

Dopaminergic pleasure is future focused. It is focused on possibility: what could be or what hasn't happened yet. It is not rooted in the actual reality of our lives. This is very different from the type of pleasure that is based in the here and now.

Thankfully, there *is* another type of pleasure that you can experience—one that is rooted in what's actually happening in front of you. This pleasure is sensory—involving what we taste, touch, smell, feel, and see—and it enables us to enjoy life as it is happening and then reflect upon it after the fact.

If dopaminergic pleasure is all about *anticipation*, this one is about *appreciation*.

TAKING IT ALL IN

Appreciation can get us off that treadmill of constantly seeking more. Down to the neurochemical level, appreciation pleasure is distinctly different from the type of dopamine rush that depends on novelty and newness. Appreciation, or experiential pleasure, actually produces different chemicals in your brain: serotonin, oxytocin, and endorphins, those naturally occurring opioids that also mediate pain and stress. We will talk more about this in the chapter on gratitude. For now, just remember that our brains look very different chemically when *we want something* from the way they look when *we are experiencing and appreciating what we have*.

Appreciation pleasure is harder to come by than the dopamine-inducing variety. This is partly due to the fact that the dopamine circuit and the appreciation pleasure circuit tend to suppress each other. According to Dr. Lieberman, "When one is active the other is more or less at rest." Don't miss this. Not only does dopaminergic, anticipatory pleasure pass quickly without truly satisfying us; it actually *suppresses* our ability to appreciate what is happening in the moment. In our "more is better" culture, no wonder that it is often difficult to stop and be present and to experience life as it is happening.

The ancient text of Ecclesiastes refers to this notion as far back as 450–200 BCE. The author of this book is unknown, but rabbinical tradition believes it to be King Solomon, who was known for his unmatched wisdom. The author of Ecclesiastes writes, "Whoever loves money never has enough; whoever loves wealth is never satisfied with their income. This too is meaningless" (5:10 NIV). A different translation of the text (NLT) puts it this way: "How meaningless to think that wealth brings true happiness!"

All I have to say is Biggie was right: mo' money, mo' problems.

Interestingly enough, the author of Ecclesiastes ends the chapter talking about how true pleasure is found in enjoying simple things: "Even so, I have noticed one thing, at least, that is good. It is good for people to eat, drink, and enjoy their work under the sun during the short life God has given them, and to accept their lot in life" (5:18 NLT). Sounds like appreciation pleasure to me.

The presence of dopamine circuits makes me think that we were indeed intended to crave more. But perhaps this "more" looks different than what we've been told: more rest, more laughter, more connection, more spirit-filling wonder, more silence, more service, more joy, more long embraces, more slow walks on the beach—more of the things that truly satisfy.

So let's be clear: dopamine, in the right quantities, is a good thing. Dopamine circuits have kept us alive and ensured our survival as a species. These circuits are constantly stimulating our thinking about what's next and what could be beneficial to us. People who have strong dopamine circuits are often visionaries and creators. Dopaminergic personalities are forward thinkers, writers, and leaders—people focused on possibility and those who bring things that do not exist into being. Yet those people high on dopamine often do have trouble living in the present and appreciating the here and now. Their minds are constantly fixated on the future, whether it involves more work, more pleasure, or more creativity. We also know that because of this, they often experience higher levels of discontent and distress.

The more that we do something—the more often we repeat a behavior—the more we strengthen that neural circuit to do it faster and more effortlessly. We create new pathways and form superhighways in our brains that strengthen that repeated behavior. As I mentioned before, our brains' incredible ability to change and adapt to our environment is called neuroplasticity. Neuroplasticity can be powerfully adaptive in that it enables humans to learn new, beneficial habits, get rid of old ones, and heal and recover from trauma. Yet this ability can endanger us as well, living as we do in a "bigger, better, and more" culture. Corporations, advertisers, and politicians constantly and *intentionally* stimulate our dopamine circuits to fire, triggering continual desires for that which we don't have.

If you have watched the documentary *The Social Dilemma*, you know that social media platforms are designed to capture your interest and keep you addicted to the content you are seeing. This includes ads that are relevant to your preferences. Have you ever been browsing for an item, and suddenly you see it advertised everywhere you are online? That used to freak me out, and I started looking behind my shoulder as if someone were tracking my every move. This is not a good look for an anxiety therapist, so I stopped. But the fact remains that our information—every move we make online—is sold so that we will spend more time on these platforms. Social media companies and advertisers constantly flood our feeds with things that we have shown interest in, such as that seaside resort or that pair of cute leopard flats.

These platforms rely on *manipulating* dopamine circuits to stimulate more desire. And exactly how much time do we spend online? Check your screen time in the settings of your phone, which will show you exactly how much time you spend on your phone and where. Companies trying to sell us things have successfully switched our dopamine circuits into overdrive. And the longer and more frequently those circuits are activated, the stronger they become.

Simply stated, the more focused we are on what we want or should be, the less aware we become of what we *already* have and sometimes even who we are.

DESIRE AND SUFFERING

The idea that the desire for more creates discontent is found in many religious traditions. The Buddhist tradition speaks of the Four Noble Truths, which are incredibly relevant in this conversation on happiness. The first truth confirms that suffering exists in our lives. No one escapes it; it is a given.

But it was the second truth that astounded me when I first encountered it. This truth states that suffering is caused by *craving*. The word for craving in Pali, a language closely related to Sanskrit, is *tanha*—which, when translated, literally means "thirst." Tanha signifies our unquenchable desire or longing for more.

The third truth states that the end of suffering happens when we can eliminate our cravings or desires. Essentially, we no longer suffer when we do not desire anything and are able to accept our lives with all of our challenges, be it an illness, an unfulfilling job, or a difficult relationship. The fourth truth, then, details the path to getting there or ending the suffering. Because of these truths, one of the main goals in Buddhism is to put an end to wanting. Buddhists fervently seek the letting go of all desire.

Perhaps you have met a person who is constantly saying, "If I just could buy a house . . ." or "If I could just find the right person and get married" or "If my kids would just listen" or "If I could just be more successful at my job" or "If we could just go on vacations like they do." Yes, it is good to have goals and dreams that motivate us to take action. But goals also have the power to direct our attention and time into achieving and acquiring. Unless we intentionally balance our goals with practices that ground us in the positive and pleasurable realities of the present, the desire for those good things can lead to constant wanting and comparison. Goal-driven people can easily lose perspective on what is good because they are already in pursuit of what could be better.

Deeply ingrained in our national roots—almost embedded in our country's DNA—is the belief that material possessions are the true measure of success and worth—a.k.a. the American Dream. But research suggests that wealth does not translate into happier people. The World Happiness Report reveals that wealthier countries tend to rank *lower* in perceived happiness and life satisfaction than less wealthy countries.

Why then, when we have so many opportunities, options, and a higher standard of living, are we so unhappy?

WHY LESS IS MORE

When I was twenty-three years old, a romantic relationship that I had been in for five years ended. A bit of a drama queen, I declared soon before the relationship's demise that if my boyfriend and I broke up, I would go and work with missionaries in some remote part of the world. Gratefully, I ended up in Costa Rica, one of the most beautiful countries on earth. My parents say it looks a lot like Sri Lanka—although most Sri Lankans say that anytime they land in a warm place with an ocean and palm trees. (Apparently, Puerto Rico, the Bahamas, and Jamaica also look *just* like Sri Lanka.)

For six months, I volunteered in a protected community for the children of alcoholics and drug addicts. The children lived in simple dorm-like homes with host families. I worked long hours with a psychologist during the day, and I spent any free time I had in the afternoons helping the kids and cleaning and cooking for them at the house. This was by no means an easy life. I got lice a few times and was bitten by bedbugs, mosquitos, and fleas so badly that I had more than one hundred bite marks on my body when I got back home.

Yet I had never been happier.

In Costa Rica, I did not want a thing.

I had no social media, which didn't exist yet. I experienced no FOMO, as I had no idea what anyone else was up to. I didn't think about what I was missing, because I was so engrossed in what was happening around me. I had no anxiety about my future; because my days were so full, I had no time to think of it.

Each morning I woke up, did a devotional reading, and asked God to help me experience the beauty around me and to be helpful to those who needed me. Every day both happened. I had a purpose, and I felt useful. The kids kept me grounded and focused, in contrast to the previous few months, when I had been walking around aimlessly, searching for meaning. And they were just happy to be with me. Those connections breathed life into my weary spirit.

I was amazed that my new Costa Rican friends, many of whom had far less than I had, celebrated what they *did* have far more than I ever had in the United States. Costa Ricans, or Ticos, are known to be happy people, famous for the phrase *pura vida*. These words reflect their philosophy of a "pure or simple life." We would translate it as "all good." In fact, Costa Rica is known to be one of the happiest countries in the world. With no army, the country spends 8 percent of its gross domestic product on education, believing its strength lies in human talent and well-being. Costa Ricans care for their environment, using sustainable energy sources, and take pride in the breathtaking landscape of rainforests, beaches, volcanoes, and waterfalls. The country also boasts some of the oldest people in the world, with a life expectancy of 78.5 years—longer than the life expectancy in the United States.

Economists believe that the well-being of the country is related to residents' strong networks of family, friends, and supportive neighborhoods. If there was one thing I witnessed in Costa Rica, it was the power of connection through celebration. Fiestas for any occasion, at any time of day, were the norm, and everyone was welcome. As I entered any home of a Tico, I was immediately offered cake, a meal, a drink, or whatever they had. This even proved true in the refugee community in which I worked for a time, where the makeshift homes had tin roofs and dirt floors. These people were poor. I do not want to minimize the impact of poverty on finding contentment. It is very difficult to feel at peace when one's basic needs of food, clothing, proper shelter, and safety are constantly uncertain. Having a level of financial security where one does not have to wonder how these needs will be met naturally lends to greater contentment. Even in spite of extreme poverty, what I witnessed in that refugee community were resilient people who loved, who shared, who thanked God for what they had, who laughed and celebrated and enjoyed the natural wonders around them. Even in unfathomable uncertainty, I witnessed moments of contentment.

Soon after I returned to the United States, I needed to buy toothpaste. I took a trip to the local CVS around the corner, where I was overwhelmed by a whole aisle dedicated to oral hygiene with what seemed like one hundred choices of toothpaste. I started to read all the boxes. *Whitening, bleaching, sensitive, fluoride, sparkles, mint, bubble mint*: it was a lot to take in. In Costa Rica when I needed something, I would go to the market, pick from one or maybe two choices, go home, and get on with my life. Five minutes tops. Do you know, I left CVS that day without toothpaste! I couldn't figure out which was best, so I picked nothing. Options can be overwhelming.

How much time do we spend overthinking things like this just because we can? How much time do we waste on trivial pursuits when we could be getting on living a meaningful life?

CULTURES OF CONTENTMENT

Just thinking of sunny Costa Rica might make you happy, with its lush landscape and tropical weather. But apparently many people living in cold Nordic countries are also exceptionally satisfied with their lives. From 2013 until today, the five Nordic countries of Finland, Denmark, Norway, Sweden, and Iceland have ranked in the top ten of the World Happiness Report. Nordic countries even occupied the top three spots from 2017 to 2020.

Knowing the sun can significantly impact mood and mental health, I have wondered how this could be true in a part of the world known for cold winters and long, dark days. Many theories try to explain why this is so. Between the extensive social benefits, the trust in their government, the equality reported between immigrants and citizens, the freedom to make life choices, or some combination of these factors, they have lower anxiety and burnout rates. Residents in these countries feel taken care of, are better connected to other people, and have a healthier work-life balance than we do in the United States. Lower stress, as you will see in part II, is a significant factor in well-being and longevity.

What fascinates me most, though, is hygge. A few years ago, it trended on social media, as everyone's blankets, candles, and hot chocolate were #hygge ad nauseam. Having originated in Denmark and Norway but now adapted in other Nordic countries, the concept of hygge (pronounced *HOO-ga*) describes an atmosphere of warmth, well-being, and coziness. I recently learned that one definition of hygge is "feeling at peace to enjoy simple pleasures of being in the moment." It might include a cozy reading nook, comfy sweatpants, a heated blanket, a cup of tea, or warm socks. Summer hygge boasts bonfires on the beach, outdoor movie nights, or delicious meals with friends and family. When it comes to cravings, I would certainly crave more of all of this. Talk about appreciating the gifts of every season!

Nordic culture is also quite clear on what hygge is *not*: hours looking at your phone, spending time isolated in your room, and *especially* not buying costly, trendy things. These life-wasting practices are not encouraged.

Hygge is considered "a defining feature" of Danish cultural identity and an "integral part of the national DNA," according to Meik Wiking, the CEO of the Happiness Research Institute in Copenhagen. Can you even imagine living in a culture that encouraged people to slow down and be content—all without buying anything to help them do so? Can you imagine what it would be like if enjoying the simple pleasures of life was woven into a nation's DNA? This is a culture that is all about appreciation happiness!

Our culture makes a life of appreciation very difficult. When our natural human desire to look for more is compounded by cultural currents and manipulated by advertisers' power, it becomes hard to discern what really matters. I'm not just talking about the United States either. Britain is just as guilty, as are many other wealthy countries around the globe. Our national priorities reflect a particular set of values, and as a result, our biology is changing to accommodate it. More desires instantly satisfied by the new and novel mean more pathways strengthened to seek it. As a result, we are paying a very, very high price with regard to our mental and emotional health.

If we want to feel different, we have to begin making different choices. This may be far harder than we realize. We will have to overcome powerful cultural forces—especially one that literally, neurobiologically programs us for discontent and insecurity. Its impact is so alarming and significant, especially when it comes to our kids, that it necessitates its own chapter in this book.

You might think that adults would be better equipped to handle this particular force, but not necessarily. I have the same conversations in my office with forty-year-old women as I do with twelve-year-old girls, all struggling with the same issues created by it.

That's right, I'm talking about social media.

Maybe we'd be headed in the right direction if we could just let go of our global obsession with . . . selfies.

CHAPTER 4

Selfies

"Ugh! Give me that!" my fourteen-year-old daughter groaned. For a second, I thought she might be passing a kidney stone. But no: it was suffering brought on by her forty-five-year-old mother's improper selfie angle.

She grabbed my phone. "Why do people in your generation hold it like that?" she asked. "That's the worst! Your forehead looks three times bigger."

Your generation? Ouch. That hit a nerve. Just that morning, at my annual mammogram, I had to check the box beside the next age group up from what I had checked last year. That's always a great way to start your day. Nothing like squinting at a white piece of paper saying "Yes, you old" right before getting your boobs squashed.

I later found out my daughter and her friends deliberately take "mom selfies"—selfies from bad angles, similar to how I was taking the photo—as a joke. For real? These kids need jobs.

According to research, ninety-three million selfies are taken *per day.* (And by the way, that number was reported from Android devices alone.) I also learned that one out of every

three photos taken by eighteen- to twenty-four-year-olds is a selfie and that some people report taking up to *eight selfies a day*.
If you still don't believe this photo phenomenon has become
woven into the fabric of our culture, get this: the use of the
word *selfie* increased 17,000 percent from 2012 to 2014. Clearly
selfies have infiltrated our way of life: what we talk about, how
we see ourselves, and also how we spend our time.

Selfies also have a significant impact on our kids' well-being.
But social media more broadly affects the moods of even the
most mentally stable adults in one way or another. What seems
like mindless or innocent scrolling through our Instagram photos or Facebook feed actually immerses us in a *disingenuous*
world that creates *genuine* discontent.

Let's talk about selfies first. Selfies are exactly that: focused on
yourself, how you present yourself, and how you will be perceived.

Research points to the evidence confirming that as a culture,
we are becoming more narcissistic and less empathic. Sure, factors other than selfies and social media are at play. Overscheduled kids are losing out on unstructured playtime—the time they
learn how to read emotional and social cues from their peers
and respond in a caring manner. During unstructured playtime,
kids *have* to develop some level of empathy if they want to make
friends in order to keep the playtime going. We live in the age of
helicopter parenting, where kids are overpraised, and every non-
achievement is medal worthy just because the child showed up.
You better believe I threw away all my daughter's preschool soccer medals. Those were the years she literally only touched the
ball when it rolled over her foot accidentally. Yet the development of narcissistic qualities has been accelerated by this form
of self-promotion, which has become almost socially obligatory.

We have research to prove that selfies have made us more selfish. An interesting study published in *Personality and Social Psychology Review* surveyed nearly fourteen thousand American college students to measure empathy in young people. This study confirmed that college students are less empathic now than students three decades ago. Each year resulted in a lower score than the previous one. In fact, the average American college student in 2009 scored as less empathic than 75 percent of students in 1979. Using the Interpersonal Reactivity Index, "empathic concern" dropped the most, closely followed by "perspective taking," which measures how well a person can see things from another's perspective. This decline in empathy also correlates with a steady rise in mental health issues for this population. This may partially explain why young adults are more self-focused: it's much harder to consider the needs of others when you are feeling anxious or depressed.

The study ended in 2009, well before the explosion of social media platforms in 2012, but from what psychologists have seen, we can safely assume that this trend has continued. We know that mental health issues in teens have continued to rise steadily. Additional studies relying on what is called the Narcissistic Personality Inventory confirm that empathy is on the decline and narcissistic qualities are increasing in this younger generation year after year.

Although psychologists don't think that social media is the sole cause of narcissism, it tends to attract people with narcissistic tendencies and strengthen those who have these qualities already. A world where you can exist as an idealized version of yourself and attract followers that validate it by telling you how amazing you are—well, it's near *heaven* for narcissists.

Conversely, social media can be used for good and can foster empathy. Social media exposes us in real time to world crises, hurricanes, earthquakes, and terrorist attacks, as well as personal hardships such as job losses, tragic deaths, and depression. We can support a vast array of organizations and individuals by donating money or even commenting to offer emotional support and encouragement. We are constantly inundated, however, with this type of information on our feeds, and many of us develop both news fatigue and compassion fatigue, as we are desensitized to the constant barrage of traumatic and upsetting news. This can adversely affect our ability to feel empathy and our motivation to take action. Bad news all the time is too much for our hearts and minds to process. As a result, many feel overwhelmed and end up doing nothing.

If we are constantly focused on how we look or what our lives are like compared to those of our friends and even celebrities, we become consumed with these thoughts about ourselves. We may have less bandwidth to think empathically about the needs and situations of others. At the same time, when everyone appears to be doing well and enjoying life—at least as seen through the lens of a curated profile—we can forget that there is another side to that story. Why would we feel empathy for people we follow on social media when everyone's lives look so perfect?

COMPARISON CULTURE 101

Have you ever taken a trip to Florida and felt pretty good swimming in your grandma's pool and enjoying the nice weather—only to jump on Facebook or Instagram and see some random person's fabulous yacht excursion island-hopping in Greece?

You might not even know this person, but suddenly the Sarasota sun and a little relaxation don't quite cut it.

Or maybe you were stuck at home on the third snow day in a row in February and saw your friend's Instagram story filled with photos of her with a drink in hand on some beach in Jamaica (#currentsituation). All you can think is *I hate you*—but you hit the heart-eyes smiley reaction. Because she *is* your friend, after all. And yes, that might have happened just this afternoon.

Maybe you have been working out, cutting back on the carbs, eating cauliflower rice every day, and feeling good about your two-pound weight loss, and then popped on social media to see your girlfriend, who apparently doesn't work out and eats whatever she wants—at least in front of you—in her sexy red bikini (#thisis40)?

These images trigger thoughts that most certainly affect our mood one way or another and ultimately affect our behavior. This pattern is the premise of cognitive behavioral therapy, which we will talk about in the second part of this book. There I'm going to show you how to use this pattern to your advantage.

Every week in my office, I hear stories of anxiety and discontent. As I dig for the details, exploring what conversations or events might have triggered feelings of frustration and negative thoughts, I find that comparison often emerges from beneath the surface. This is no surprise. Comparison has always been a frequent flyer in sessions, and I have come to recognize it as a usual suspect.

Comparison is not something I take lightly. I know of its potential, and it is dangerous. It has the power to highlight our innermost insecurities and create tension where it hasn't existed.

Most of all, it leads us down a path of deep discontent and toward a focus on what isn't instead of an embrace of what is.

SHOULDING ON YOURSELF

That's right. Don't do it. You heard me. Don't *should* all over yourself. Because that *should* gets messy, and you're the one left to clean it up. Often that cleanup gets passed down to those closest to you too.

I should be in a different place than I am right now. I should have a baby by thirty-five. I should be able to provide more for my family right now. My kids should respect me more. I should be making more money. I should be more successful. My child should have done better in school. I should be happily married by forty.

We constantly *should* all over ourselves, and comparison, so readily accessible at our fingertips, tends to be the catalyst. *Shoulds* are birthed from expectations that come from society, from people we know, and from ourselves.

No one knows this better than women, especially if you are South Asian.

South Asian aunties, particularly Sri Lankan ones, can be ruthless. One good thing (I guess) is that you never have to wonder what they are saying about you behind your back because they just tell you to your face. Once, at a family birthday party, an auntie spotted my cousin and me and made a beeline for us. With an astonished look on her face, my aunt exclaimed to my cousin, "Lakshmi, what happened to you? You're fat!" In that moment, I silently gave thanks to God for the parasite I had gotten from a girls' night out in the city that left me nauseous every night and unable to eat much for months.

These aunties are known for asking other questions—ones that leave us vulnerable and exposed. Even if you haven't been blessed with such an auntie, these types of questions, or variations of them, may still permeate your life: "Why aren't you married yet?" "Why haven't you had a baby yet?" "Why haven't you found a good job yet?" We actually ask them of ourselves, as we see others meeting these expectations when we're not.

Careful, though: *shoulds* can lead us to do things that we may know in our gut are not right for us. We're simply driven by the pressure to meet the expectation. Many times I've seen women *should* all the way to the altar. I remember one of my clients bursting with excitement with her engagement news. As she showed me her ginormous, sparkly, emerald-cut stunner, she told me she had met her fiancé six weeks earlier. That seemed more than enough time to get to know someone at her age—or so she thought. This thirtysomething bride was well aware that her biological clock was ticking. She was the last to get married of all her friends. She was tired of cotton candy–colored bridesmaid dresses and bachelorette trips to Miami. It was *her* time now.

From the moment I met her, I heard her *shoulding* left and right. "For God's sake, I should be done with birthing babies by thirty-five, not just starting the process. I should have been married years ago. I thought I would have been . . . I'm attractive, I'm Ivy League educated, and I make six figures. I shouldn't be single at thirty-five."

Apparently, she thought a few sessions of premarital counseling would make up for the quick trip to the altar, and so she brought in the lucky guy. Carefully, I tried to squeeze in some observations that this beautiful but incredibly different pair were, well, incredibly different—like blow-torch-and-ice different. My thoughts, though, were quickly deflected by stories of their passionate, dopamine-charged sexual chemistry. (Well, they didn't really say that exactly, but you know what I mean.) Unfortunately, that marriage ended three years later, after two beautiful kids and with four broken hearts.

Shoulds can be useful if we use them as red flags. When we identify a *should*, we can stop and ask ourselves two powerful questions: "But what do I need?" and "What do *I* truly want?"

My accountant, Stacy, once told me she was advised that she should have over two million dollars to retire well. A strong, tough woman who had emigrated from Greece, Stacy didn't buy it. "No, I don't!" she told me in her raspy voice. "When I retire, I can eat bread and feta and tomato salads in my village in Greece and be perfectly happy." If only we stopped once in a while and considered what it would really take to be content, we might uncover a desire that is free of expectation and full of attainable truth.

Sometimes we *do* find truth and life and even happiness in the *shoulds*. When what we think we should do aligns with what we believe to our core, we can find contentment and joy when we attain these types of should goals. However, I encourage my clients to replace the word *should* with words like *want*, and the truth still remains without the same pressure: I *want* to spend more time with my kids. I would *like* to see my aging parents more often. I would *love* to keep my house more organized (a girl with four kids can dream). It sounds different because we have released the urgency and pressure and changed our perspective. We have unearthed and extricated our *own* desire from the expectations. This change in phrasing also makes room for those things in life that prevent us from getting to that goal. Those unexpected life events are normal, and they never pay attention to a well-planned timeline. Changing the language allows us to speak to ourselves with understanding and empathy, and that helps us move on toward our goals.

Social media does not discriminate in the comparison game. We have avenues to compare virtually everything: from our kids to our cars to our homes to our bodies. *Especially* our bodies. For women in particular—especially adolescent girls and young adult women—a constant visual diet of manipulated images of near perfection is costly. The price we pay, literally, can be thousands of dollars. Even more disturbing, striving for this type of perfection can cost one their life.

Want proof? Buckle up.

INSTAFACE

A couple of years ago, I came across an article in the *New Yorker* that described the Instagram face, or Instaface. This face would look very familiar to you if I included a photo. The author, Jia Tolentino, described it as a "cyborgian face": both human and synthetic, where human parts are altered to exist in an environment different from a normal one. The face is youthful, with doe eyes and long eyelashes; high cheekbones; poreless skin; a tidy, neat nose; and thick, full lips. Then there is the expression. Tolentino writes, "It looks at you coyly but blankly, as if its owner has taken half a Klonopin and is considering asking you for a private-jet ride to Coachella." Pretty much sums it up. And trust me, I know what half a Klonopin looks like.

This doctored-up face permeates our social media feeds. Many social media influencers' faces now resemble Tolentino's description of a cyborgian face through the use of filters and even plastic surgery. This composite look has become the unnatural and yet widely sought-after standard of beauty.

The article describes the Instaface as featuring an "overly tan face, South Asian influenced brows and eyes, African American influenced lips, a sharp Caucasian nose and a cheek structure that is predominantly Native American and Middle Eastern." Tolentino writes that it's as if everyone looks like they are descendants of Kim Kardashian and Kendall Jenner (who also kind of look like each other). Over the past few years, I've had a harder time recognizing if someone is a person of color on social media and sometimes in real life. I now find myself constantly saying, "Wait, I thought that woman was white, but now she's Black?" Many people on social media look like they might be of mixed race. Yes, the multiracial population is growing annually, but I realized my confusion was in part due to Instaface.

It is fairly easy to attain this look on screen through the plethora of filters available—which, by the way, is favored by the algorithm. Better algorithms translate to greater exposure and more validation on Instagram. Filters on each platform, in addition to widely used apps such as Facetune and BeautyPlus, fix jawlines, brighten eyes, plump lips, and even thin out thighs instantly.

But this isn't where it ends.

Plastic surgery—especially noninvasive procedures like fillers and Botox (hand-up brown girl emoji)—has become as common as going to the gym for those who "take care" of themselves. Famous plastic surgeons on social media boast literally millions of followers, including celebrities ready to shout them out like a five-star Yelp review for Chinese takeout. According to the American Society of Plastic Surgeons, Americans in 2019 spent more than $16.5 billion on cosmetic plastic surgery and minimally invasive procedures. What does it say about our culture that more than 90 percent of these procedures were performed on women? The messages are loud and clear, and it's women who are hearing them.

Plastic surgeons now report that it is very common for women to ask to look like how they do through their favorite Instagram filter. In fact, the 2017 annual survey of the American Academy of Facial Plastic and Reconstructive Surgery found that 55 percent of surgeons reported having patients request surgery for the purpose of "looking better in their selfies." That's compared to 42 percent the year before. In 2021, we know even three-year-olds know how to take a selfie, and the average patient is also getting younger and younger. More than 70 percent of facial plastic surgeons reported an increase in these procedures for women *under thirty years old*.

For the right price, fantasy truly can become reality.

If you have had any of this kind of work done, you know it ain't cheap. "Just a little bit of Botox"—most women's gateway drug into the cosmetic world—can cost upward of $2,000. This now seems to be the normal or at least accepted price of self-esteem, confidence, and ultimately happiness.

WARNING: OBJECTS IN THE PROFILE ARE DIFFERENT THAN THEY APPEAR

I have friends I've gotten to know through social media but not in person. They might be a friend of a friend, and we had heard about each other and so decided to connect. I only know these friends by their photos. Given everything I just said in the last few paragraphs, this can be problematic.

I once attended an event at our local playhouse, and a woman walked up to me and said, "Hi, Niro!" I think she could tell from my polite but vacant smile that I didn't recognize her. I squinted and tried to connect her face with some memory but came up with nothing. But a second later, my big Sri Lankan brown eyes—which give away everything—must have widened like saucers as it occurred to me who I was talking to. This was the first time I had ever seen her in person, and she looked nothing like the photos she had posted on social media. This woman looked at least twenty years older than all her profile pics, which were a *bit* more than filtered. Girlfriend had some sort of time-machine app.

I decided right then and there that all my busted, just-woke-up-in-the-morning photos, taken from the "mom selfie" angle my daughter warned me about, had an important place on social media. I'd much prefer people be pleasantly surprised rather than shocked when they meet me in real life.

Not to go all Carrie Bradshaw on you, but in this culture of #blessed, what really is the ratio of harm to good when it comes to social media? Do the filters really make us feel better about ourselves? Do our altered images make us truly feel more confident?

The research says *not at all.*

A 2018 study published in *Body Image Journal* revealed that women who posted selfies reported feeling more anxious and less confident about their appearance than women who did not post selfies at all. The kicker here is that the women who could retouch and retake their selfies prior to posting felt *equally* anxious as women who posted the first take of an undoctored image. While you might think an image of yourself that you are happier with would have a positive impact on self-confidence, it's apparently not the case.

These researchers from Canada and Australia demonstrated that in the act of posting a selfie, you begin to evaluate and scrutinize your appearance. As you modify the images through filters and apps, you become hyperaware of your perceived imperfections and flaws. The more photos you take, the more imperfections you see and the more anxious you feel. This is often the manner in which women trigger feelings of self-objectification. We begin to treat ourselves as objects valued merely for our appearance rather than whole human beings.

This became an issue for me when I began to bring my therapy insights to social media. When I posted photos, I started to notice that my nose was bigger than I thought it was. It had always looked fine to me, but as I started to post more, it started to bother me. When I was a child, kids would make fun of how big my nostrils were, saying that a train could ride through them at any moment. My response usually was "The better to smell you with—and you stink." (Which was a total lie because to this day, I have the worst year-round allergies! What's the use of a big nose if it doesn't even work?) Yet I started to analyze my appearance more often, especially as I started to do television interviews. I would literally cringe to see myself on camera.

I started to research makeup contouring methods to make my nose look smaller. That didn't seem to help much, so I actually began to consider rhinoplasty (because who really wants to say "nose job," especially when you are writing a book). I researched the recovery time, side effects, and cost and viewed an excessive amount of images of people who had done it. At the time, I was a forty-three-year-old, happily married mother of four, who was well educated and ran a successful private practice. Remember, other than a few times as a kid, I had never really been bothered by how my nose looked until I started to see myself frequently in all types of media.

In the end, I decided not to go through with the procedure. A few of my children have noses that look like mine, and I do not want to send them the message that any of theirs need the slightest bit of alteration. Ralph Waldo Emerson's words—"What you do speaks so loudly that I cannot hear what you say"—often come to my rescue. I want my children to know that they are beautiful just the way they are, and I do not want to cast any doubts that would make them think otherwise.

That moment of realization was enough to put things in perspective for me. After a few more weeks had gone by, I also realized that it was actually the close-up images of myself—the selfies—that had created my discontent. I eventually learned to say to myself, "Honestly, who the hell really cares what my nose looks like?" I couldn't believe how much Instagram, which I had considered an insignificant app, had significantly shaped my self-perception. I couldn't believe how much of my time those thoughts had consumed.

My nose and I are all good now. I take Zyrtec every day, and it works well enough. And I'm back to seeing myself the way I want to see myself: as a not-perfect, whole, beautiful human being defined by many more significant things than my nose. Many women have a hard time getting to this place, and I still need reminders some days. If there is one thing selfies take very well, it's our perspective.

THE PRESSURE OF PERFECTION

If you are a young woman between the ages of sixteen and twenty-five, still developing your sense of self while spending, on average, five hours a week on social media uploading and posting selfies, it's hard to stay confident. Several studies have confirmed that simply posting selfies leaves women more vulnerable to clinical eating disorders and anxiety disorders.

When I was younger, I may have seen a waif-thin model on a television show that I could only watch at the time it aired or in the pages of a magazine that arrived once every couple of months. But now girls are flooded daily with images on their phones of perfect bodies: posed, filtered, and edited. These images have become their standard of worthiness. I cannot overemphasize the perpetual mental distress this causes. When girls reach for their phones several times an hour, the impact these images have on their self-perception is significant.

This is exactly what I meant by the cost often being life itself. We know that eating disorders have continued to increase and begin at younger and younger ages. Eating disorders are the third most common chronic illness among adolescent females in the United States. We take this very seriously in therapy. Anorexia is considered the most fatal mental illness, with a mortality rate of 10 percent. One in five anorexia deaths is due to suicide. The cost is very, very high.

MIDDLE SCHOOL: SAY NO MORE

If I asked you if you wanted to go back to middle school, I'm pretty sure I know what the answer would be. Most of you reading this book didn't have the constant barrage of perfect images to make your awkward-looking thirteen-year-old selves feel worse. And thank you Jesus for that, because adolescence was not kind to me. I was overweight; had brushed-out, curly hair that looked like an Afro (beautiful if you are Black but a little strange on a twelve-year-old South Asian girl); and wore thick, black, Sylvia Weinstock–esque glasses. One day a wise orthodontist—oblivious to the plight of the totally awkward—slapped headgear on me too. So I might as well have just called it a day for the rest of middle school. Oh, and the yearbook staff misspelled my name in the yearbook that year: "Nirdo," which, read out loud, was "Nerd-o." You can't make this stuff up.

These days, my middle school daughter, Natalia, has my sixth-grade school photo saved on her phone. I was posing in what I thought were the coolest acid-washed jeans; I remember thinking I looked great that day. Of course, my daughter and her friends think it's hysterical. *I think seeing what I looked like at their age makes them feel much better about themselves.* I'm glad I can serve that purpose. (By the way, I showed that same picture to that same daughter when she was five years old and asked her if she knew who it was. She didn't hesitate for a second. "Uncle Rahul!" she exclaimed confidently. Need I say more?)

Aside from the awkwardness of middle school, many of us vividly remember the friend drama. Was this girl really my friend? If so, why didn't I get invited to that party? Why didn't she tell me what that other girl said about me? So much drama! Although it looks different for boys, they, too, have their emotional ups and downs and struggle with self-confidence. We who are parents get to relive all of this now as our kids experience this tumultuous stage of life. Lucky us.

Honestly, I'm so grateful my most awkward days were not documented and posted for the world to see for years to come. I'm relieved that all I really have left now are a few photos that are only in my possession. I'm glad I never knew how many parties I was not invited to because I didn't even know that they happened. Ignorance might not be bliss, but it is certainly less stressful.

This, however, is no longer the case.

Social media is the reason I have the same exact conversations with married women with two kids as I do with twelve-year-olds in therapy. Photos of a fun girls' night out that you didn't know about until you saw the post? Why would your friends post it if they knew they didn't invite you? Or maybe it was a playdate with your closest friends and their kids—except you and your kids weren't invited. Did you do something to offend someone? Were your girlfriends texting about it on a group text you weren't on? Was it that harmless comment you made that night out for drinks or at your friend's birthday?

And here is where we question the truth of our experiences, because what we see does not align with what we thought we knew. *I thought we were great friends. I thought they cared about me.* We begin to overthink instead of communicate, resulting in more stress and anxiety. We might even feel we have lost our place of belonging, one of our deepest insecurities. Yet we forget we are often seeing or hearing only one part of the story. This is the danger of constantly comparing our real lives to a curated one.

From the most mature adult to the angsty teen, social media has an impact on our mental health and therefore on our happiness. It can cause us to question our reality, our ability, our appearance, and our worth. And constant scrutiny, whether it's our life or someone else's, takes us quite far from contentment.

Even the strongest of relationships are not immune from the impact of comparison and expectation. Our relationships could be perfectly fine or at least good enough. Yet this type of pressure can even create trouble in what seemed to be . . . paradise.

CHAPTER 5

Paradise

The *New York Times* ran a story in 2019 with the title "Honeymoon Hashtag Hell." The article described one couple's wedding bliss turned honeymoon nightmare. The husband, Mr. Smith, recalls the picturesque sunsets not with fondness but because "it was like a photo shoot for a magazine that would never exist." His new wife worked in digital marketing and disclosed that she had to "prove to the world that [she] was having a great time." She did admit that she noticed her husband was unhappy but did not allow this detail to ruin her mood—just so she could attain her coveted photos. The couple recalled that much of the trip was spent trying to catch the sunsets, posing for the perfect photos in freezing waters as the sun went down, and then spending hours shooting more pics, editing, and planning Instagram posts.

This scenario is actually rather common these days as family and friends track couples on their honeymoon with the expectation that they will detail their often extravagant and dreamlike adventures. Expectation once again leads to pressure. Many feel the need to prove their honeymoon is as worthy as the relationship itself. Or perhaps it's the reverse—the relationship is only as worthy as the honeymoon. Between researching the best food items that would photograph well or the prettiest beach, the Smiths did not have much time to connect in paradise. The couple nearly separated upon their return.

Few of us live out our relationships on social media quite to the degree of the Smiths. And I don't know how many of us would actually call our romantic relationships "paradise." But we know from the research that relationships may be the most important determinant of our well-being. Whether it's friendship, romantic partnerships, or parental bonds, our strongest emotions are often evoked through relationships. If you are in a romantic relationship, the person you spend the most time with will have a significant impact on your feelings of contentment.

Because of the busyness of modern-day life, the pressures to succeed, and our need for validation, daily time to connect with loved ones is hard to come by. When we do find time, many people feel exhausted and turn to mindless scrolling or binge-watching a show instead of meaningful connection. One is easy and accessible, and the other requires effort and energy. Many people also feel more validated by their "followers" than their true friends and family. Oftentimes, these followers are people they don't even know with whom they don't have a real relationship. Real relationships are hard! Phones provide an ever-present distraction that comforts tired and weary minds on many levels.

You may be thinking there is too much emphasis on social media in this book. But we have to talk about social media here as well, in a chapter about our relationships. It is a serious force that impacts not only our perception of our relationships but the relationships themselves. Discontent easily creeps in when we begin to compare the quality of our own significant relationships to the curated images of the ones on display.

ARE YOU SLEEPING?

I'm asking you this to make sure you are still with me but also because I often wonder about this. Have you ever seen photos on social media of a couple sleeping, only to realize that one of the "sleeping" people must be holding out the camera? Or maybe it's a photo of a couple's romantic Valentine's kiss—yet one of the kissers is simultaneously photographing that supposedly intimate moment. Maybe you are drawn into that fairy tale at first—but then, if you're like me, you realize what's going on and think, *Wow, that's so fake!*

Thousands of these types of photos are posted every day. These kinds of photos promote a relationship culture that is anything but authentic. A 2017 study, published by the National Institutes of Health, revealed that people generally thought their own photos were authentic but perceived other people's photos as disingenuous and even narcissistic. Some 82 percent of people reported that they were tired of other people's selfie-type photos but that they themselves posted their own up to seven times a day. Clearly there's a disconnect between our self-perception and our perception of others.

It's almost as if it being disingenuous gets rewarded. There you go, 250 likes later (even if many of those likes come from people thinking the same thing as me). Here we are, trapped in this game of "I'm going to pretend this photo of you is great, but that's not what I really think." This then sends the message "You are awesome; keep doing this." This ultimately continues this disingenuous cycle of validation.

A distorted reality creates distorted perspectives. On the surface, this may not seem like a huge problem. But deepening the disconnect of a device-dependent, already disconnected culture has tremendous consequences. When the gift of support is beautifully and meticulously wrapped in duplicity, we have reason to question the validity of many things, including our own relationships.

CRAZY IN LOVE OR JUST CRAZY?

My husband, Ed, is not a social media guy. He rocked his Myspace, checked that box, and was done with it all. Sometimes I watch him, his readers on and brow furrowed, repeatedly tapping his phone and asking questions like "How do I see who messaged me?" and "Where is my profile?"

Yet one year on our anniversary, Ed decided to *stand up* on Instagram and declare his love for me. His first-ever IG story featured photo after photo of our wedding and other milestones, accompanied by captions such as "Love of my life." I saw the Instagram story, and although it was very sweet, I came home wondering what the heck had happened to my husband. "Are we OK?" I asked—because, one, we don't do this publicly and, two, I have incredibly biased theories about people who do.

Love-declaration posts to significant others make me cringe. Some are witty, short, simple, and sweet. But the ones that make you feel like you accidentally opened someone's mail and read their secret love letter—those I just can't take. This is one of the drawbacks of being a therapist. When people think we are psychoanalyzing them at a cocktail party, we aren't. (I mean, unless your behavior is making *everyone* wonder what's wrong with you.) But sometimes we do read into things more than we need to. I wonder when I see these posts, *What made this person write this for everyone to read? Shouldn't this message just be written in their birthday card? What are they trying to prove to themselves, to their partner, or to the world?*

I know—so judgy, right? #therapistsissues

But over the years, I have seen many couples for counseling who I know have serious, deep relationship issues. Sometimes they haven't slept in the same room for years, or one is thinking of leaving the marriage, or one has had an affair—just to name a few. Oh, and the amount of anxiety I have seen when someone finds out their partner is following the infamous ex after some high school reunion—well, let's just say it's enormous.

Social media, though, is an alternate universe. I have seen couples scream at each other on my couch, uncertain if they should stay together—and then the next day on Facebook enjoying a glass of wine and frolicking on a mountain like the von Trapps in *The Sound of Music* (#drunkinlove). Deception shrouded in perception: there is a lot of that when it comes to what you see about relationships. Perhaps it's not as serious as deception, but certainly there's more to that story than that one perfect, meticulously filtered moment.

Again, we may not be as dramatic as the honeymooning Smiths, but most of us have seen the impact of our cell phones on our relationships. Whether it's scrolling on social media, answering messages, or browsing the internet, I have seen the destructive impact of all these apps on relationships—my own included.

IT'S A FAMILY AFFAIR

"Get off your phone!" my kids and husband often scold me. It's more of a joke now, but at one time, it wasn't. Between hosting a podcast and sharing helpful therapy tips, I once spent a lot of time creating content and "connecting" on social media. I was not aware, however, just how much time this took until I noticed how my family began reacting to me. Although my family insisted I spent a lot of time on social media, I was certain I didn't . . . until I realized I did.

Very few of us can post and walk away. We check comments and likes, comment back, and then check again. Remember that hit of dopamine we receive when we get new feedback in the form of a comment or like? So naturally, we keep doing it . . . and then lose track of time. Sometimes *a lot* of time. While I'm on there, I might click on a "quick recipe" or "quickly check in" at a store I like. One click leads to another and there goes 45 minutes in a blink.

Kids pick up on this right away. Many articles have detailed kids expressing to their teachers their frustrations with phones. *USA Today* quoted a second-grade girl saying, "I don't like the phone because my [parents] are on their phone every day. . . . I hate my mom's phone and I wish she never had one." The journal *Child Development* published a study suggesting that restlessness and anger outbursts in children are related to "technology-based interruptions in parent-child interactions." One thing I remember growing up was that when my mom didn't listen to me, she was usually busy doing things around the house. She never ignored me repeatedly because she was staring into a device, constantly consumed by something more interesting that didn't seem all that important to me. You can see how this could incite considerable anger in kids. For many, this pattern has become their normal.

Kids may not always have the language to express this discontent, but one thing I know is that our spouses certainly do. As we were getting ready for bed one night, my husband turned to me and said, "I'm jealous of your phone." I quickly brushed it off with an awkward laugh. "That's crazy," I said and looked away. He continued quietly, but I could tell he was mad: "I wish you would spend even half the time you spend on your phone with me."

I knew he was right. My phone, not my family, had gotten some of the best hours of my day. At this point, it had become the third person in our marriage, and it was affecting my kids too. I knew that I had to do something about it. If this is you too, hang tight. In part II, when we talk about what you can do about this, I'll tell you the rest of the story.

The night my husband brought up this issue, I remembered the photo essay "Removed" by artist Eric Pickersgill. He shot photos of people holding their devices in everyday life situations. We see images of families out to dinner, neighbors celebrating at a barbecue, and couples cuddling on a couch. He poignantly captures couples in their wedding attire, sitting atop a decorated car with "Just Married" written on the windshield behind them, and even couples in bed together, much like my husband and I were that night when he confronted me. Yet what we see in these photos is that not one person is looking at the other. Everyone is staring into their devices.

But here's the catch: Pickersgill photoshopped everyone's devices *out* of the pictures. Where their cell phones used to be is just empty space. So essentially, everyone is looking at nothing. People are simply staring into air, their bodies curled around air, their hands holding air. Their faces are devoid of expression, and though in the company of many others, each individual seems solitary. All of them miss the beauty of their surroundings and the people in them.

Pickersgill's statement on our interpersonal disconnect and fixation on devices could not be clearer. He told the *Washington Post*, "I'm not trying to tell others what to do with their time, I'm just hopefully offering up a moment of realization. I just personally need the reminder to put it down because it is an addiction."

Connection is the life force of our common humanity. It enables us to simultaneously express emotion and feel it, to give and to receive. In a few chapters, we will explore even more about connection and how it is found at the heart of contentment. Devices, most definitely, are the number-one modern-day threat to our ability to experience it.

RELATIONSHIP GOALS

I know you've seen #couplegoals by now. Don't get me wrong, I enjoy a good hashtag. But we might subconsciously begin to measure our relationships against a standard that might not be what we want or need. We often lose sight of our partner's or our kids' strengths if we are measuring them up to someone else's. Once again, comparison enters the picture and can distort our reality rather quickly.

It's easy to get swept up in wanting what we don't have and then feeling pressure to get it. As I have mentioned, wanting often prevents us from both recognizing and savoring what is already good in our lives. But the worst thing I've experienced when I am fixated on what I want rather than focused on what I have is regret—both in the moment and years later.

We had looked forward to Ed graduating from his orthopedics residency for six years so we could finally have a "normal" family life. Residency is hard on relationships. Young doctors are overworked, exhausted, and poor and just trying to get to the finish line. What they don't tell you is that when you do, life isn't that much easier. New doctors can look forward to the worst call hours, the lowest salaries in the practice, and a gazillion dollars in student loan debt kicking in.

After his residency was over, we still didn't have the life I had imagined. I had spent the last six years dreaming of a house in the suburbs with a big yard that my kids could run around in. We certainly couldn't afford that yet. I wanted our family together on holidays, having dinner around the table—not visiting an on-call room. Although my hardworking husband was doing everything he could for our family, he secretly felt awful that he could not provide what I wanted. My expectations, unbeknownst to me, created pressure in our marriage. I have since learned that many men struggle with feelings of inadequacy in their relationship for the same reason. As far as I was concerned, this was not what was supposed to happen after residency. We *should* have been at a different point in life. We *should* have been like everyone else: raising families in their happy homes, creating beautiful childhood memories. There I went, *shoulding* on my whole life!

As a therapist, I often help my clients try to appreciate the good in their situation rather than solely focus on what could be better. But I had a hard time doing that myself during those years—and there was *so* much good. Instead, I remember wondering when we wouldn't be in so much debt. I remember wondering what other people would think when they came to visit us in our condo—Would they assume we were not successful?—and explaining to them why we weren't living in a house.

And you know what? No one cared but me. Absolutely no one.

This happens far more often than we realize. We look for validation not in *our own* truth—those things we hold sacred—but in the *perceptions* of other people. The crazy thing about those years was that I was looking to see if other people *thought* we were fine, well, to decide *if* we were actually fine. Yet if I had tuned out the noise of the expectations and the *shoulds* and listened to that still, small voice underneath, I would have heard the truth: we were exactly where we were supposed to be.

Twelve years later, the landscape looks different. I am grateful for our life together every day, but I know it comes at a cost, as you read about at the start of this book. Our relationships often pay that price. I now know that none of what I had so longed for brings the type of happiness I thought it would. I am also well aware that it could all change in a heartbeat. One devastating phone call. One momentary bad decision. One natural disaster. One diagnosis. Nothing material can ever make up for certain types of losses.

But that younger me was looking for validation that I was OK and seeing material success as a measure of worth. Big mistake. Huge. I wish I had shopping bags to hold up, ironically. (Channeling my inner Julia Roberts.) That kind of happiness just doesn't run very deep. I have worked with plenty of successful people and celebrities who literally have everything they could ever want and can buy the rest. They live glamorous lives and appear to the world to have it all together. But many are still searching for happiness, for worth, for identity, and for purpose. Those who have managed to find contentment within the culture of affluence have grounded themselves in the practices and perspectives we'll look at in part II.

The depression and anxiety fairy doesn't skip over people who can check the money, power, and success boxes. If that were the case, we wouldn't see such high rates of addiction and harmful self-medicating behaviors in affluent populations. In fact, we know that children who grow up wealthy experience symptoms of depression and anxiety at rates three times that of nonaffluent children. They are also two to three times more likely to abuse substances, creating a toxic, self-destructive cycle. And as my wise mama reminds me, "You are only as happy as your unhappiest child." If you have ever had a child self-harm or become addicted to a substance, you understand *every* relationship in the family becomes devastatingly affected.

Looking back, I wish I could tell my younger self to drop all that comparison baggage. It prevented me from seeing the most precious gifts I had right in front of me. Gifts like moments with the most inquisitive, wide-eyed toddlers who adored me and a low-maintenance home that afforded me the time to do so. Days where it only took a sprinkled ice cream cone and a story snuggled under a knit blanket to make them happy. Evenings when I'd walk in the door from the office and have six little feet race toward me to see who could wrap my legs in a hug first. Looking at how fast my kids are growing up, with two taller than me already, I think of how much more I could have enjoyed those relationships had I been more present in my real life rather than in the life I thought I should have had. Those are moments I can never get back now, but they certainly can teach me how I want to move forward.

SO WHERE DO WE GO FROM HERE?

I think it's pretty clear by now that the issues that prevent us from feeling content are deeply intertwined with the culture that we have come to accept as normal. There are aspects of it that we readily consider desirable. But as I have asked before, Is the price tag worth it?

I want you to know that therapists are worried right now. When therapists are worried, um . . . worry. We've seen a *lot*, and it takes a lot to shake us. The cultural factors that create pervasive discontent are powerful. Although we as adults are affected by them, we have a point of comparison, remembering what life was like before. We remember what it means to live more simply with fewer distractions and can try to get closer to a life like that. This constant striving for more—this validation-seeking and comparison culture—is the only air our kids have been breathing since day one. There is no other normal for them unless we create one. Looking at the state of our collective mental health, we know we cannot afford not to.

We need to rethink *how* we want to live what poet Mary Oliver calls our "one wild and precious life." Stress, anxiety, depression, self-medicating behaviors, and the physical manifestations of all of these: these are the result of how we are doing life right now. So I ask you, Are we really living the way we were intended to live?

People, creating a culture where we are healthy, peaceful, and content necessitates change. We have got to change our habits.

We have got to begin asking questions about what we value and if our lives truly reflect those values. Living healthy lives requires us to look at our real priorities—meaning how we spend our time, money, attention, and energy—and see if they align with the things we hold most sacred. When we begin to align how we live with what we value, we begin to change the culture around us and find peace within us.

Culture is the atmosphere in which we live. It is the soil that surrounds us and gives us life or drains it from us. Our current culture is very good at nurturing seeds of discontentment, which can grow swiftly into something we no longer recognize as our own life.

As you read in the preface, my husband and I found ourselves in this place not too long ago. The good news is that *our* collective soil—the heart and strength of what *we* are made of—is always fertile ground for new growth.

Lasting, sustainable change happens one small step at a time, day by day, month by month, until we normalize a new thing. And this new thing will be woven, slowly and intricately, into the rich, magnificent fabric of who we are and how we do.

OK, let me keep this real.

In the world we live in, our quest for happiness will never end. Happiness is transient and will never fulfill our deepest longings. We gravitate to things the world says will make us happy because they also validate our worth. Yet the fact that we even need to validate our worth is at the heart of the problem and the reason we will constantly keep searching.

We have the opportunity to experience something more profound than happiness, something with more staying power that promises us a life of calm, peace, and well-being. If we embrace the life we have right now and the gifts we have already been given, we have the potential to live a full, meaningful life. Very simply, this is a life of contentment. In part II, I am going to show you how to find it.

Can this type of switch happen? Can we move away from the endless pursuit of more to living grounded in the idea that we have enough? Yes, most definitely. But it might look different than you think. Again, it's one small change and then another. I've seen the transformative power of a process that respects and acknowledges that which is small and consistent. If one person commits to this process, then it has the potential to impact another. If a few people commit, then we may transform a family. If one family commits, then we could influence another, slowly leading to a community.

Creating healthy communities requires a cultural shift that will take time, education, and the investment of many families, communities, and organizations. But thankfully you don't have to wait until then. You and your family can experience moments of what I'm talking about right now.

I need to talk about one more thing before we get into what you can do to find contentment. Anytime I help a client make healthy life changes or whenever I start down a new path that helps me evolve into a stronger and more truthful version of myself, a phenomenon occurs. This phenomenon is going to happen every time you move toward a better version of yourself or to a new level in your life. You are guaranteed to encounter obstacles, roadblocks, and setbacks. It may even feel like the whole universe is working against you.

That's probably because it is.

CHAPTER 6

Habits

I love a little drama. This is probably why I became a therapist. I'll get to the whole universe-working-against-you bit in a
moment (and no, this is not a conspiracy theory, so relax). All
of that will make more sense if you understand how habits level
up our purpose in life and can lead to a life of contentment.

Most of your life is made up of habits you don't even notice.
You wake up in the morning, and most of you check your phone
first thing. (Statistically, we know this.) You walk into a room
and turn on a light. You get hungry and head for the kitchen.
You tie the same shoe first every morning. (Yes, that one surprised me too.) You brush your teeth before you go to bed. You
fall asleep in your child's bed after reading a bedtime story in
the workout clothes you wore all day, makeup on and contacts
still in. (OK, maybe that's just me.) But really, according to
the *Journal of Personality and Social Psychology*, 43 percent of
everything we do in a day results from our habits. What's even
more interesting is that we perform these actions while we are
thinking about something else.

You might not think of some of these behaviors as habits, but
they are. We have programmed them into our brains through

repetition, and they meet an important need or craving. We have a craving to find out new information in the morning that pertains to us, so we check our phones. We crave food, so we go to the place where we can find it. We crave sleep, so at night, we get ourselves ready to go to bed. Cravings and behaviors go together. As we saw in an earlier chapter, research suggests that if the behavior is rewarding—meaning it enables us to satisfy the craving—our brain remembers it and creates a pathway for it. The more often we do the behavior, the stronger the pathway becomes, until we no longer even have to think much about it.

How much more content would we feel if we would automatically do the things that make us feel calm? What if we could create habits that wired us for contentment? The good news is we most certainly can.

This link between cravings, behaviors, and rewards is important when we think of creating a new habit. Again, we have to do the new thing consistently enough to build up the pathway to the point where the habit becomes second nature. If we can't do it consistently, the pathway will become weaker, and we will end up giving up on whatever change we hoped to make. New weight loss and exercise regimens—especially drastic ones that are too hard to sustain over time—are great examples of habits that often fail for this reason. When we start a new practice, we want to make it as easy as possible.

WHAT YOU DON'T KNOW *WILL* HELP YOU

We know from research that we can do certain things to help make a new habit stick.

Make it easy. Making the new behavior as easy as possible means we can sustain it over a long period of time. This includes anticipating some of the things that cause us to give up.

Say I want to start working out in the morning but haven't been great about this in the past. I know I usually hit the snooze button, go back to sleep, and then miss my window of time, and it's over. This particular issue is one that I have struggled with, so I had to come up with some strategies to help me overcome it. Now I start getting ready for my workout the night before. I set my alarm across the room so that I have to get out of bed to turn it off. I pick out my workout clothes and put my sneakers near my bed. I also decide which workout I'm going to do before I go to bed: walking, high-intensity interval training, or strength training. Do you see how we can make it easier to even start a behavior with a little planning? We can eliminate any potential situations that might prevent us from doing what we set out to do.

A year and a half ago, I began a six-week workout challenge. We were at what we hoped was the tail end of the pandemic, and I had picked up my share of pandemic pounds. (Note to self: do not leave a bag of dark-chocolate peanut butter cups on the counter, ever.) I found that I was able to stick to the workouts six times a week, which I have *never* done in my life. I began to think about why this worked when other types of challenges didn't for me.

What I realized was that this challenge had all the components of successful habit formation. The classes were convenient, offered in person and online several times a day, so I could always get to one. The workouts were short and easier than I was used to, so I didn't feel the mental resistance I would if I had to motivate myself to do something hard. I also prepared the night before, as I described, so I didn't have to think much when I woke up.

I also signed up for this challenge with a few friends. Accountability and support are gold when you start something new. According to studies, if you can find someone who shares similar goals and can join you on the journey, you are *twice* as likely to achieve them.

Connect it to something you already do. We have to pick the right situation or environment to facilitate the behavior. This means connecting our new habit to something we already do regularly every day—something that we don't have to think about. My workouts happened every morning within one or two hours after I woke up. Since I designated the approximate time of the workouts, I signaled to my brain that waking up and working out go together.

Make it rewarding. We have to make any new behavior rewarding. The practice has to effectively meet a need that we have or provide a noticeable benefit. My new workout routine was effective in part because it was rewarding. I had more energy during the day after I worked out, which helped me with my demanding schedule. This energy elevated my mood, so I felt happier and calmer—a benefit we know comes from exercise. I also connected with friends during that time, which was both enjoyable and motivational. When rewards involve connection with others, they are next-level satisfying.

Rewards run deep when it comes to habit strength. Sometimes a behavior itself is rewarding, like having a glass of wine with a good friend. Sometimes we have to *create* the reward, be it emotional, mental, or physical. Research suggests that if we can evoke an emotion alongside the reward, our brains will remember the behavior as *even more* rewarding. When the brain is rewarded, it remembers the action and encodes the message "Whatever just happened, do it again." This might sound familiar to you from an earlier chapter: our reward neurochemical, dopamine, is at play here. The brain is designed to remember useful, rewarding behavior, and this is how a habit is solidified over time.

As I mentioned before, we create and strengthen neural pathways as we introduce and repeat new habits. These pathways form a loop that involves the craving and the behavior to satisfy the craving. Think of the *reward* as that one piece that closes the loop and solidifies that pathway. Essentially, the reward seals the deal.

Rewarding yourself for a new habit might be as simple as saying out loud, "That was great!" when you choose the apple over the donut. You might think to yourself, *Well done, you fabulous thing*, when you take a deep breath instead of reacting aggressively in an argument. Cheer for yourself like a helicopter parent cheering on the sidelines for their child's mediocre athletic ability. Even if it's not a big deal, do it! We have research in cognitive behavioral therapy to prove that it makes all the difference.

At the end of each chapter of part II, you will find a "Turning the Key" suggestion, which is one small way to begin your practice of creating a life of more contentment. At the end of each directive, I suggest you tell yourself something positive, like those encouraging statements above, or that you simply smile to elicit positive emotion.

This idea of reward is in no way to minimize the frustration, sadness, or anger you may be feeling. That would be considered toxic positivity. I suggest saying positive things to yourself or smiling as a way to create a psychological reward. Smiling reflects a principle in dialectical behavioral therapy called opposite action: a behavior that encourages someone to act in a way that is *opposite* to whatever overwhelming emotion they are feeling.

I like using smiling for a couple of reasons: First, when we are doing something hard or feeling frustrated, forcing ourselves to smile or even laugh can seem so crazy that it actually breaks the cycle of negative emotion when we feel stuck. Second, we usually don't realize how much tension we are holding in our bodies at any given time, especially in our face, which has forty-two muscles. When I remember to smile, it always helps me relax, even when I'm feeling the most intense. Sometimes it evokes a memory or makes me realize I do have things to smile about, even when I am feeling negative. Smiling tends to release that tension both physically and emotionally, as it helps connect us to something positive. There is solid research behind this! The next time you are ready to quit in the middle of a tough workout, or angry at the person who cut you off on the road, or tired of hearing your kid call your name for the one-thousandth time, just try it and see what happens.

Habits make our lives far easier than they would be if we had none. We don't have to make decisions about the hundreds of daily tasks we have to do in a day; we just do them. Then we can expend that neural energy on other, more difficult processes that require it. Those more difficult processes include engaging in the practices that help us experience full, contented lives; impact others; and even fulfill our purpose. See why I said habits help us level up? So it is 100 percent worth it to invest the energy in creating helpful ones. You've got more important things to think about!

These keys to contentment are *not* items on a to-do list—though they are things to do. These keys are about the transformation of your identity and the lens through which you see and experience the world around you. This is soul-healing work. This is life-giving work. It will affect you and everyone with whom you come in contact. Your life literally depends on it.

So given all the potential of habits to change your life, you may begin to see why forces bigger than you might take notice when you move in this direction . . .

RESISTANCE AND ROADBLOCKS

In therapy, my clients and I come up with plans that will help them heal or achieve the goals they desire. We strategize about those obstacles that might prevent progress. We discuss strategies that will help them advance toward their goals or toward healing. But if we don't talk about resistance and roadblocks—both internal and external—they can take us by surprise. When we can anticipate the obstacles, plan for them, and figure out how to circumvent them, we see transformational change.

Before you begin any of the practices suggested in part II, I want to make sure you can identify forms of resistance and know what you can do to get past them. And because we are about to embark on a journey that involves growth and change, we can know there will be resistance. This resistance might come from ourselves, or from family members or friends, or sometimes from the universe itself. We can do a few things to outsmart it.

Steven Pressfield, author of *The War of Art*, describes resistance as a force that "obstructs movement only from a lower sphere to a higher. It kicks in when we seek to pursue a calling, or evolve to a higher station morally, ethically or spiritually." Because you also have great power to influence the transformation of others as you gain new habits, I would bet my entire career on the fact that you are going to experience resistance. If you don't know the saying "New levels, new devils," you are about to see it firsthand. Personally, I take these unexpected challenges as confirmation that I'm on the right path, exactly where I need to be in that very moment.

Let's look at two types of resistance to change: internal and external. Both attempt to stop your progression. Both require some sort of response.

THE WAR WITHIN YOU

Internal resistance includes the things within us that prevent us from moving forward. Some may describe this as negative self-talk: negative messages that appear to come from ourselves. Self-sabotage—behavior that undermines what we truly desire—can also be a way we experience this war within.

But even though this resistance *seems* as if it is coming from you, in your own voice, it is not you. One of my clients tells me she sometimes wakes up in a funk, full of this kind of resistance. "She's *back*," she says, referring to the negative and toxic thoughts she experiences. My client is right: our negative thoughts are not us. They do not reflect who we truly believe we are. But they can be pretty powerful in convincing us otherwise.

I have identified three types of internal resistance—I call them the three unwanted visitors. Think of them as those houseguests who come for an obnoxious amount of time, don't help at all in the kitchen, expect to be fed for days, and then don't take the hint when it's time to leave. While they may overstay their welcome, they can eventually be shooed out of your house and be sent home.

Visitor 1: Self-doubt. These are the thoughts we have about ourselves that prevent us from believing we can do whatever we are trying to do. *I'm not good enough. I don't have enough. I don't make enough money to do this. I'm not smart enough.* Psychologists call these "limiting beliefs." Anytime you are moving to a higher level, self-doubt is common. You may even find that you experience what's called *imposter syndrome*: the sense that you don't deserve to be at this new level, whether it means at a job, or in a social network, or even sharing the truth of your new experience. Almost every successful person I know has experienced imposter syndrome at one point or another.

A quick aside: if God or the universe brought you to that point, you better believe you deserve to be there and that you have been given what it takes to make it. If you didn't belong there, the way would not have been made. Self-doubt seriously impedes our ability to reach goals and can often bring the process to a screeching halt. It's important to talk back to this houseguest with this truth as soon as you see him.

Visitor 2: Fear. As an anxiety specialist, I could write an entire book about fear. Many of us could, actually, because fear is so common these days. Therapeutic approaches offer countless ways to deal with fear and anxiety. For now, though, I just want you to be aware and notice fear when it shows up in your house. Be sure to red-flag what-if questions and worst-case scenarios. *What if I take this step and I lose everything? What if people think I'm an idiot? What if I have regrets after I make that choice?* Negative thinking always adds another layer of resistance that we have to power through. When we consider those questions while feeling fearful, we go to answers that usually aren't very helpful.

If this type of thinking is familiar and seems very normal to you, you may have had anxiety for a while. If this is the case, therapy is absolutely worth a try. I love treating anxiety because with the right research-based tools, it can be managed and even cured. You can be free from anxiety to experience your life in all its fullness. It takes work, but it can be done, and recognizing this type of negative thinking is the first step.

Visitor 3: Unbelief. This one is for you people of faith—those who believe there is a higher power working on our behalf. You believe in God, or the universe, or some power that helps direct you on this path of life. You might even believe that along this designated path, you will find your purpose.

You've seen evidence in your life to support this belief, but there are times when you stop believing. You start doubting that what you have experienced is true. You doubt that you were put on this earth for a purpose. You doubt that a divine hand is guiding your steps and interactions. For the person of faith, unbelief can be devastating because it shakes the foundation of what you hold most precious and true. When we fall prey to unbelief, we can lose the inner strength and courage needed to do the hard things that fill our lives with meaning. We begin to doubt our voice of wisdom and our ability to receive wisdom as well. Unbelief might even cause us to give up on the goal itself.

Let's be clear: all three of these unwanted guests are liars. They lie to you about yourself, about your capabilities and situations, and about the beliefs you hold most sacred. Sometimes the lies are the same and just morph into different versions depending on the circumstances. In that case, "new levels, *same* devils" is more accurate.

What should you do about these unwanted visitors? Kick them out yo' house—like out the front door. I will talk a little more in detail in part II about how to manage some of these thoughts, but for now, DJ Jazzy Jeff them.

We have evidence in cognitive behavioral therapy that if we *externalize* these thoughts—that is, if we recognize them as voices separate from our own—we are better equipped to stop them. Then we don't run into them as often. You do realize your resistant thoughts aren't paying rent to live in your house, right? So they don't deserve to occupy that space. Less time thinking these thoughts prevents us from developing neural pathways that strengthen them and give them more power. And you thought I just liked the Fresh Prince.

STAYING STRONG WHEN THINGS GO WRONG

I'm sure you've had your own run-ins with Murphy's Law, the universal truth that states that if something can go wrong, it will. Is it just me, or do you find that Murphy's Law shows up at the worst possible times too? You misplace your keys only on the day you are running superlate to work. Your child gets sick only on the day you planned to finally get together with your best friend for lunch. You spill your coffee only on days you decide to wear white. Some of these events are just those everyday obstacles that are a part of life. Some, however, almost appear intentional in the way they prevent us from moving forward in significant areas of our lives. Obstacles and challenges appear out of nowhere.

That's what I faced the day I locked myself out of the house. I have never experienced more resistance to moving forward in my purpose than I have when writing this book. One weekend, I left my family at home for a quiet weekend at our beach cottage, where I get major work done. Uninterrupted moments are few and far between for this mama of four. I can only liken it to pumped breast milk: you don't waste a drop.

By Sunday afternoon, having made great progress and having found my flow, I decided to take a short thirty-minute break. I left the house quickly to meet up with my friend Lena to take a walk, during which we chatted, relaxed, and became inspired by spectacular glimpses of the ocean. Upon my return, I realized I had left my keys *inside* the house. Luckily, I did have my car key. I knew that the property manager for this house didn't live far away, and I hoped she could loan me a house key. So I called her—only to find out she had moved an hour's drive away. My thirty-minute break now turned into three hours of precious time wasted. On top of that, I hadn't eaten anything that day and now was good and hangry. (Not to mention that it was Sunday, so Chick-fil-A wasn't even open!)

Often in the exact moment we are doing what we feel called to do, we experience resistance. I have observed this phenomenon time and time again. I now look at resistance as an indication that what we are doing is important and of great value. This realization has helped me put the roadblocks in perspective and carry on.

External resistance can also come in the form of distractions. Don't I know about this one! I'm trying to convince my favorite psychiatrist that I have ADD, but he won't buy it. As I wrote this book, I found myself looking up just about anything online—from Target curtain rods to the best recipe for triple chocolate cake—right in the middle of researching neural feedback loops. Distraction serves as a very real type of resistance today; our devices now provide endless opportunities to be distracted everywhere we go.

So now this is where it might get a little woo-woo for some of you, but just hear me out. As a person of faith, I think some external resistance is the same thing Christians call "spiritual warfare." Just as we believe in an omnipotent force for good (God), we believe in forces that oppose this. You certainly don't have to be a Christian to believe in an enemy or in dark spirits, of sorts. When we are talking about a meaningful life, one of peace and purpose, we are talking about living exactly the way God intended us to live. And I believe forces are trying to prevent this kind of awakening and evolution. When you are content, full of peace, and living a life of purpose, you become quite a force for good in this world. Recognizing this type of resistance is half the battle, as it can be extremely deceptive and easy to get sucked into. It can take the form of any of those lies our three unwanted visitors tell us, and it can even shape-shift into some of those unexpected and challenging life situations.

Now I'm not suggesting that you call *every* obstacle spiritual. I kind of hate that. Locking myself out of my house is not the devil; it's my own absentminded fault. Let's not give the devil all the credit for what we've rightfully earned ourselves. That scenario, however, could have been an opportunity for me to get negative, frustrated, and off course—and *that* could have been real enemy territory. Our unfortunate situations, big or small, have the potential to be used for good or evil around us or within us. We can often make the choice to allow one or the other. When we know how to cultivate calm, we have the bandwidth to stop, think, regulate our intense emotions, and find perspective. When we can do this, we grow in character, patience, and perseverance.

ALL GREEK TO YOU?

If this particular spiritual stuff doesn't resonate with you, you might identify with a different type of spiritual warfare as a way to explain resistance. The ancient Greek philosopher Plato speaks of the war within through the analogy of a charioteer who rides a chariot pulled by two winged horses. He explains that the human soul, or psyche, is made of three parts: one part represented by the charioteer, and the other two parts by the two horses. One horse is dark, wild, almost deaf, hard to control, and mortal. (Why is it always the *dark* one? Just sayin'.) The other horse is white, noble, and well behaved; it responds to direction and is immortal.

The charioteer and his winged horses—again, the three elements of the soul—are headed toward the ridge of heaven, where they will find the things our soul longs for: beauty, justice, courage, and wisdom. If they get there and can see the "essence" of these things, they will nourish the horses, who will then stay in flight. Yet there is a battle to get there, and the charioteer is constantly moving up and down, struggling to control these two powerful yet opposing beasts. The dark horse, representing hedonistic pleasure (of course), wants to pull the charioteer back to earth. The white one, symbolizing honor, strains to move upward, toward those noble things in heaven.

There is so much more to this analogy, but we can use it to describe the internal warring of the spirit. All of us have a carnal side that craves an excess of pleasure in many forms, be it food, wealth, sex, or other things. It's not that these things are bad at all, but the cravings for them can overtake everything else we know to be good in life. We often refer to these as the "desires of the flesh," which battle the higher, spiritual side that seeks the more noble virtues. It is often an internal battle—one filled with resistance. This, too, is spiritual warfare.

One more word about resistance. Because I do believe in a God who wants us to live a life of contentment, peace, and purpose, I don't believe resistance just happens *to* us—I believe it happens *for* us. Resistance is one of the greatest facilitators of our growth. When we take the steps to recognize it and overcome it, we grow stronger, wiser, and more assured. I have seen in my life that everything has worked together for my good when I have chosen to adopt the perspective that it can and will. So depending on your perspective, yes, the universe may work against us, but it also works very much for us.

Hopefully now that you know a little more about resistance and roadblocks, you can identify them as you begin to make changes in your life that will lead to more peace, calm, and fulfillment. If you recognize resistance in your life, take it as a message that you are on the right path. I have come to believe the greater the calling, the stronger the resistance. So if that's you, carry on, friend. You are exactly where you should be.

CHOOSING CONTENTMENT

In case you haven't figured it out by now, I don't have the "secret" to calm and purpose. Many of the eight keys to contentment we are about to explore you have already heard about and may be practicing. If so, I hope you see them through a different lens or are moved to think more about them. Even if you make *one* small change that helps you find peace and perspective and if you go back to it again and again throughout your lifetime, this book will be a win-win for both of us.

Over the course of fifteen years as a therapist, I have noticed that certain clients work through issues faster than others do. Some clients move through issues fairly quickly; others have a harder time moving forward and get stuck. Part of what we do in therapy is help people get unstuck. Yet as much as I try to move them along—giving them tools and exploring the issues—the decision to move forward always lies in their hands, not mine. Some experience more resistance, both internal and external, than others. I'm not saying that everything is a choice. We often suffer the consequences of decisions made for us without our permission. Your path to finding contentment might be strewn with rocks and debris.

Mine was not. I came from a family with two married parents who sacrificed a lot for me and my sisters. We were deeply loved, affirmed, and provided for. This made all the difference in my core beliefs about myself and my ability to find the good in any circumstance. And yet as a young adult, I had my own struggles: developing my identity as a woman of color in white environments, suffering from pervasive anxiety, and even experiencing clinical depression for a time. Yet I also had support that I could always come back to. For this reason, some of these things have been easier for me to adapt than they might be for you.

Still, I know—and every piece of research confirms—that regardless of your past or present challenges, you can find contentment. Through years of patient interviews, I have seen that we still have the power to make choices. We are capable, and we often underestimate the power of our own agency found within. We need to tap into this.

Contentment is a choice we make. It's a choice we make to willfully live life in a different way—a way, as you have seen, that is very countercultural. We have the choice to adopt a different perspective when we consider what is best for us and our families. We have the choice to engage in practices that may seem unfamiliar or uncomfortable but have been proven to give us more of what we are longing for.

Most of us feel overloaded with information, and no one needs even one more good tip if it just creates more stress in their life. Everyone these days—or so it seems—is a therapist or life coach or has some helpful advice to empower you to "be your best self." As you begin this next part of the book, start small and make whatever first steps you choose to do *easy*. You can certainly build up to more once it is wired in your brain, but do not underestimate the power of the small. Also, focus on only one or two new changes at a time. Too many too fast just won't stick. A small change here and another one there add up to more collective calm.

When I begin anything—be it writing my first book or starting yoga—I often get intimidated by the people who have been doing it forever. (Like people who have actually worn yoga pants to a yoga class and not just to the grocery store.) Yet I always go back to the verse from the Hebrew Scriptures: "Do not despise these small beginnings" (Zechariah 4:10 NLT). It is the small changes that actually lead to real transformation because we can make them consistently. This is how we fight resistance: that small change takes that first step on this path to finding true contentment.

But spoiler alert: there is so much to be found on the journey—so much to take in and experience, so much that is satisfying and full—that you might just forget you were searching for something in the first place.

Please recognize that contentment does not happen overnight. Be patient, and know that failure is accepted and welcomed here. All of these things you will read about can be thought of as practices. We need time to wire the concepts into our brains. Each requires repetition, some degree of consistency, and a whole lot of choice making. *This is why a book alone will never make you happy.*

But we aren't here to talk about happiness, right? What we are about to uncover is far more powerful than that.

PART II

The Eight Keys to Contentment

CHAPTER 7

Acceptance

I'll never forget taking Carolina when she was three to her pediatrician, who happens to be my mother. This fourth child of mine has proven to be the most strong-willed, feisty rule unfollower in our house, with an unshakable confidence that forty-year-old women envy.

My mom asked how things were going at home—as if she didn't already know. I love how she pretends we are real patients. "Well, we are having a hard time getting Carolina to listen when we say she can't do something," I said. I was hoping saying it out loud in front of her Amamma might motivate Carolina to think about this.

"Carolina," my mom said, looking up from typing her notes, "why don't you want to listen?"

Carolina, who had been crinkling the tissue paper on the exam table, looked straight into her doctor-grandma's eyes. Without missing a beat, she replied, "Because I want what I want."

Isn't that the truth.

Whether we are talking about changing a tough life situation, interacting with a frustrating person, improving parts of ourselves, or starting a new habit, we tend to focus on what we want—or, perhaps, what we didn't get. We want what we want.

Practicing acceptance is probably the hardest of the eight keys to contentment. That's why I'm starting with it. In terms of finding contentment, it is by far one of the most important habits. We can apply this practice to tough life situations, parts of ourselves we struggle with, and the difficult people in our lives. Acceptance also enables us to separate what we *want* from the reality of what we actually *need*. This vital process is the gateway to finding contentment.

What we want and what we need: many of us don't stop to differentiate between the two. We are led by strong feelings and urges that are hard to dispute. Yet when we can't change a situation or person, fixating on what we want and often can't have leads to more frustration, stress, and—get this—*even more wanting*. This pattern creates palpable discontent and distress in our lives. We easily lose focus on what is good and what is working for us. In fact, the research illustrates that people who do not practice acceptance, in some form, experience decreased life satisfaction. They also experience higher rates of anxiety and depression in comparison to those who do. These findings are not surprising, as resisting situations that can't be changed leads to a flood of negative emotions. Constant negativity and frustration will color the lens through which we see the world, and these emotions will certainly prevent us from seeing much good.

WHAT DO YOU *REALLY* NEED?

When one of my clients is stuck in a situation in which acceptance could provide release, I run them through an exercise. My twenty-nine-year-old client Siena felt stuck as she tried to manage some new stressors that had appeared in her life. Young, ambitious, and hopeful, Siena and her husband had been trying to get pregnant for the last few years without much luck. In addition, a recent unexpected situation at work had caught her off guard and left her feeling demoralized.

In the middle of the session, I interrupted her (which, by the way, therapists should never do) and asked, "Siena, what do you think you *need* to be happy?"

She immediately responded, "My husband and my family."

This surprised me. Given the conversations we had had about the stress of the fertility process, I was sure a baby would be on that list. "OK. What else makes you happy right now?"

She paused and considered this, and then she said, "This might sound silly, but after watching *The Gilmore Girls*, I had always wanted to live in Connecticut—and, well, now we do. I made that happen. And I love my home." She and her husband had recently moved into a house in Connecticut, which was the first they owned as a couple. "I'm really proud that we own our home."

"As you should be," I said. I kept pushing. "Anything else on that list?" I was fishing for the baby answer, but I didn't get it. We moved on to talk about what she *wanted*. That list consisted of a few items: more confidence and respect at work and more time for family . . . but still no baby.

Having run out of all my sneaky therapist tools to elicit a response, I said, "Well, we've been talking about your attempts to get pregnant. So which side does the baby fall on: want or need?" I could see the wheels turning.

After a deep silence, Siena said, "Need." I knew her pretty well by now and was aware of the things she struggled with. I wasn't sure this was her final answer.

Especially because she hesitated, I probed a bit more: "What if I said I could move you and your husband to a private island—just the two of you?"

She quickly interjected, "Sounds amazing. When can I sign up?"

"So then if you were on the island, would the baby be a want or a need?" I pressed.

She didn't hesitate. "A want. I guess it *feels* like a need because that's what everyone is expecting from us now. Everyone I know is pregnant, and I feel like we should be too. I feel like I am letting everyone down. But if it were just us? We would be totally fine on that island drinking margaritas."

Say what? Sign me up too.

Pressure. It's that complicated. Here you see my client *shoulding* all over herself because others are *shoulding* on her too. *Shoulds* make it hard to differentiate between a want and a need. This external pressure then becomes internalized. Guilt and frustration and the need to please create intense internal conflicts. Sienna is by no means alone. Many women in these situations, especially when talking about infertility, experience moments with those three unwanted visitors: self-doubt, fear, and unbelief. They hear them say things like "What's wrong with you? It must be your fault—perhaps it was something you did. Everyone else has no problem with this." These toxic mantras create another layer of resistance on top of an already heavy situation.

Having a child can absolutely fall on the need side of the list as well. I'm sure if you asked me in my early thirties, it would have. This story is not to suggest that it shouldn't. At some point, Siena's want might become a need too, and then perhaps our conversation would move in a different direction. But right now, for Siena, pressure and expectation add more distress to a time that is already incredibly painful and stressful. The pressure can prevent us from seeing that right at this moment, we might actually have what we need to be content for now. Differentiating between a want and a need is an essential step to practicing acceptance in the present moment.

As I was writing this book, my colleague Lisa (who I also refer to as my work wife because owning a business together is as close to being married as it gets) popped over to my house to bring me the latest issue of *Psychology Today*. "It's about your book!" she exclaimed in disbelief as she handed me the magazine. Well, not quite, but the cover story was indeed entitled "The Good Enough Life," and it was about finding contentment in the life you have now. I even told my husband that I wish *I* had thought of that title for the book. (Talk about wanting what you don't have.)

I began to flip through the issue, and immediately the comments on the first page from the editor in chief, Kaja Perina, got my attention: "Acceptance is not acquiescence," she writes. "Acquiescence is quiet, desperate defeat. Acceptance is the ability to distinguish between a want and a need, and to abjure the former."

Perina goes on to talk about her husband's desire for fast and fancy cars. Yet upon further reflection, she writes, he usually acknowledges that owning them would be more of a bother than a benefit. She continues, "Acceptance sheds the need. Acquiescence is not wanting to let go of the need and doing so only reluctantly."

Her insights could not be more spot on. Acceptance is powerful. It is not a whimpering resignation or a kicking-and-screaming resistance to a fate or situation that is beyond our control. In fact, it is quite the opposite. When we practice acceptance, we step into our own power. We recognize that in situations that often make us feel helpless, we have choices. We decide to no longer let an emotion, a person, or a desire control us. We put ourselves back in the driver's seat. Acceptance is the intentional release of layers of resistance that often keep us stuck in mental mud.

HOW DO WE PRACTICE ACCEPTANCE?

Acceptance is a hard concept to describe. It is often easier to talk about acceptance in terms of what it isn't rather than what it is. Dialectical behavioral therapy highlights a helpful principle called *radical acceptance*, which means a full acceptance with mind, body, and spirit. Radical acceptance is usually applied to situations beyond our control and involves some of the following self-talk.

Accept your circumstances for what they are, not what you want them to be. This means facing reality with statements like "My child is sick with a serious illness" or "I lost my job after ten years with this company."

Recognize what is in your control and what is not. "I cannot cure her or take away this illness, but I can research the best possible treatments and read books to her, play with her, and hold her to comfort her" or "I cannot get this job back, but I can devote time and energy to researching a job that might even be better for me, and I can connect with people who might be able to help me."

Suspend judgment: no should've, could've, would've thinking or self-criticism. This involves stopping thoughts that sound like *I should have known. I should have been more aware. I'm the worst mother* or *I should have worked harder. I'm no good at this.*

Acknowledge the facts of the situation to move closer to reality. Sometimes a statement like "I don't like it, but it is what it is" can help with accepting the part of the situation you cannot change.

Normalize emotions and allow for them. This means telling ourselves, "I'm going to feel sad and frustrated and scared at times, and that's OK. This situation is hard. The feelings will come and go. I will also feel strong and brave at times too."

Acceptance can look different depending on how difficult the circumstance is. In some situations, we can get to acceptance soon, and in other situations, it takes much longer. Some of my clients have wrestled with really hard things—I mean, *really* hard. Losing a young child, discovering a spouse's affair, mourning the untimely death of a parent, being diagnosed with cancer: the list goes on.

If you are struggling to accept a situation like this or even one that is more common, know that it is perfectly OK. People often feel that if they accept such tragic events, they might lose their connection to their loved one. Or they feel that acceptance means condoning or absolving. Rejecting the situation is a very normal response to trauma and grief. We don't want to believe it happened and feel that acceptance affirms it in some way. Let's be clear: you cannot bypass emotions of fear, anger,

●

or despair and go straight to acceptance. The quickest way *to* acceptance is to actually go *through* those emotions. Many of my clients who have experienced traumatic events eventually do come to their own place of acceptance, but it takes time, and often some level of healing must come first.

Again, acceptance is not saying that what happened is OK or that we are happy about it. We don't go through tragic loss and think, *It's fine that I lost my mother to cancer. I'm fine. It's fine. Everything's fine.* Or if we do, that's not the kind of acceptance I'm talking about. Acceptance is simply coming to terms with the fact that it happened; it is not avoiding or denying it emotionally. It's allowing yourself to sit with the pain, observe it, and experience it so it is easier to release.

BUT WHY ME?

Let's talk about why questions. Asking why questions is understandable, yet these questions can keep people stuck: Why did this happen to me? Why is this not-so-nice person living their best life while I'm going through this? Why didn't I see this coming? Perhaps your why questions go even deeper: Why is there so much suffering in this life? Why do bad things happen to such good people?

Why questions can torture us. They are agonizing. Honestly, I don't think we will ever have the answers to most of them this side of heaven. Even if we did, I'm not sure the answers would be good enough for us right at this moment.

For why questions, acceptance involves normalizing the asking. We accept and affirm that feeling frustrated, angry, or devastated is expected and normal. Acceptance means recognizing these questions emerge from those convoluted layers of emotion. My sister, pediatrician Dr. Krissy Satchi, when going through her own fertility journey, disclosed to me that it has been a life lesson in acceptance. "It's knowing that it's OK to feel everything you are feeling," she told me. "It's OK to feel angry or sad or resentful. You can't help it—you feel what you feel. You need to make room for that. But then you learn what to do with those feelings. You don't suppress them, because it only makes things worse. Once you acknowledge them, you can release them so you don't sit in the negativity."

That which you resist persists.

If we suppress pain, we tend to off-load it in other ways. Pain always finds a way out. Often we take it out on the people closest to us. Think of pushing a beach ball underwater. You can hold it down for a while, but in a moment, the pressure can send it flying upward, spraying everyone within reach with a force equivalent to the one you exerted to keep it down. (And I think that one sentence was the entirety of what I learned in two years of college physics.) Suppressed emotions work in much the same way.

WHEN THE BODY SPEAKS

Suppressed emotions often manifest physically in the body. Not all physical pain is the result of emotional or mental distress. But we are unbelievably integrated beings—emotional, mental, physical, and spiritual. So when one area suffers, it more than likely impacts another. Stress triggers an inflammatory response in the body, which you will hear more about later. So it's not a leap to see the correlation between the emotional and the physical. Body pain often is the alarm alerting us to pay attention to what is going on deep within us.

A client of mine, Christine, who was a busy nursing student, once came to our session complaining of wrist pain that was a ten out of ten. She was accustomed to chronic wrist pain, but in the few days prior to our session, it had gotten exponentially worse. Her pain meds, which usually provided relief, failed her. We went through the basic checklist of what could have made it worse—excessive use, a new injury, a recent viral illness—but came up with nothing. Only once before had she experienced such severe wrist pain—years ago, during a very stressful period of her life. In a seemingly unrelated vein, Christine knew she was in a relationship that needed to end, but she was having a hard time accepting it. Through the course of that session, we talked about what she truly wanted in a partner, and Christine came to accept that this relationship was not the right one for her. She decided that she was going to end it the following day.

Christine texted me a few days later, relieved that she had the courage to end the relationship. When I asked about the wrist pain, I received one word back: "Gone." Her pain had entirely disappeared, and she had complete relief for a few weeks. It has been years since that incident, and it has never again returned that intensely for her. Moral of the story: when the body speaks, stop and listen.

ACCEPTANCE ON THE BRAIN

The term *experiential avoidance* describes our choice to avoid instead of accept distressing emotions and experiences. Research strongly suggests that experiential avoidance correlates with a higher incidence of depression and anxiety in addition to a wide range of other psychopathologies. In fact, a study performed on people who practiced acceptance found that their symptoms of depression and anxiety *decreased* even in the face of stressful, negative emotion–inducing tasks. The same study also found that rumination—perseverating on negative thoughts— also decreased when people practiced acceptance. It seems paradoxical that if we *allow* for negative thoughts, we will have fewer of them. But this is exactly what the research confirms.

One study out of Harvard revealed that people who did *not* practice acceptance had decreased regions of gray matter in their brains compared to people who did. This indicates that there is less tissue available to help process emotions and stress. The same study also found less tissue in the parts of the brain stem that help process stress and anxiety in those who do not practice acceptance than in the brains of those who do. The brain has plasticity, however, meaning it responds to our changing environments and behaviors. By practicing acceptance, we can actually *reverse* this process of decreasing tissue. Come on! Is this not amazing? We can actually do things that build up these emotion-processing regions so we become more adept at handling stress and difficult life situations.

Sometimes we don't accept difficult emotions because other well-meaning people don't allow us to. Have you ever been going through something hard and had someone say to you, "Everything is going to be OK," or "It's all going to work out," or even worse, "Everything happens for a reason"? Even if you believe one or all of these, you likely don't want to hear it in the midst of frustration or grief. If you are anything like me, you may have the overwhelming urge to punch those people in the face. (I know: maladaptive coping, but oh so gratifying.) When someone minimizes your pain like this—no matter their good intentions—that person is revealing their own discomfort with uncomfortable emotions. Those simplistic platitudes offered are not for you; they are for themselves.

Rather than minimizing someone else's pain because we are uncomfortable with it, we can work to hold space for them. That means we let them feel what they are going through and support them in it so they can work their way to acceptance. In that way, we give them space for healing on the emotional level—and, as we can see in the research on gray matter, the neurobiological level too.

When we can make room and meet our own and others' pain with empathy, we get closer to releasing pain and moving forward. What people *really* need is for their hurt to be *heard* so it can be *healed*. We can then make statements to others and to ourselves (yes, talk to yourself) like "You've been going through a lot. I'm sorry this has been so difficult" and "I wish there was something I could do. Is there anything I could do to help you through this?" Such statements decrease the resistance that stands in our way of healing. Acceptance is the cornerstone of holding space for tough emotions.

Once we have acknowledged those emotions that keep us stuck—want, sadness, stress, or frustration—we need to figure out what to do with them. What *not* to do with them is also important—we shouldn't punch people in the face. If you are struggling, you may be short with your kids, so perhaps take a quiet walk alone instead of engaging them. Take deep breaths and imagine releasing all your emotions into a vast, infinite ocean, watching them drift into the horizon. This is only one strategy—there are many to help practice acceptance. You have to find the strategies that work best for you.

At some point, I try to move my clients from why questions to what questions. What can I do to help me feel better? What does this mean for my life now? What is one step I can take to move forward from this place?

Sometimes who questions can help too. Who do I know who has gone through this? Who can I talk to who will understand or at least listen? When depression hits, one of the first tendencies is to isolate and withdraw—which, as we'll learn in a few chapters, is the worst thing we can do. We were never meant to bear our burdens alone.

Answering these questions might require help from a trusted friend, family member, or therapist. It can be hard to find answers ourselves when we are wrapped up in the whys and might need support. I encourage clients to write the answers to these questions on a sticky note and put it in a place they will see every day. Then we can focus on them repeatedly.

Here is a truth you will need for the rest of this book: what we think about will grow stronger. This mechanism works both for us and against us. If we choose to focus on anxious thoughts, our pathways for anxiety increase and get stronger, and we become more anxious. But we can reprogram the default switch to something that can empower rather than victimize us. I love how James Baldwin describes, in essence, practicing acceptance by coming to terms with what happened: "The victim who is able to articulate the situation of the victim has ceased to be a victim: he or she has become a threat." As he so beautifully described, acceptance frees us from pain and enables us to step into power.

LOVE YO' SELF

Since I have discussed social media and comparison culture and their impact on our self-esteem quite a bit, we have to spend some time talking about the power of accepting ourselves. Very simply put, if we are constantly looking at ourselves through a critical lens, acceptance becomes quite a challenge. Usually we have inherited that lens from someone who was critical in our life during our formative years. Self-criticism is high-octane fuel for insecurity and self-doubt.

Now let's think about this in the context of social media. Those who aren't able to accept themselves and who critique every imperfection—physical, emotional, or behavioral—search for validation for these attributes somewhere. According to S. Carson and E. Langer, these folks "tend to be very needy and may devote considerable attention and resources to self-aggrandizement in order to compensate for perceived personal defects."

Notice they say "self-aggrandizement," which means we make ourselves appear greater or overpraise ourselves. What better place to do this than on social media? There's that cycle again: the need to validate insecurity, which fuels the need to continue the self-aggrandizement through creating a facade. All of this results in a disingenuous universe where no one knows what's *really* going on inside.

If we learn to practice *self*-acceptance, we will begin to forge a new identity—an identity in which our worth is not derived from comparison. When we don't need to look to what others think of us to get a sense of who we are, we are practicing self-acceptance. We learn to sit with the feelings of discomfort about ourselves and accept that they are OK. We learn to acknowledge the true reality of who we are, unfiltered, and we learn to find beauty in our own DNA, unique and specific to only one person and one person alone.

When I was sixteen years old, my cousin John said to me, "The most important thing you can do is to be the best Niroshini [my whole name] you can be. No one else can do that." I have spent thirty years thinking about those words. What is it that only I can do? Who is it that only I can be? Sometimes that has meant being the best wife I can be—which means being a *different* wife than my stay-at-home mom friend is. Sometimes it's being the best mom I can be—which is a *different* mom than my friend who loves crafting. Sometimes it's being the best therapist I can be—which is a *different* therapist than a friend who has been practicing for thirty years. It also means being the best me I can be by treating myself with kindness and love. And let me share with you my new definition of *best*: it is simply being the most present. I have found if I can be fully present in each of these situations, what my "best" is becomes very clear.

Acceptance means saying to myself, "It's OK if you look different or sound different or can't do what she does like she does." This last one has been incredibly important for me as a young woman of color growing up in predominantly white environments. I had to accept that I would never be like everyone else and had to find beauty and strength in my differences. Acceptance is the choice not to sacrifice ourselves on the altar of another person's identity. We all have our different strengths. What might be hard for me may be easy for you. Yet I may have strengths you don't have. When we constantly strive to keep up with someone else, we can easily lose our identity in the process. Acceptance is also the choice not to sacrifice ourselves on the altar of perfection. Nothing has been more freeing to me than making the choice to be "good enough" some days. I love reminding myself, "Whatever it is, it may not be perfect, but it is certainly good enough."

BUT WHAT ABOUT ANNOYING PEOPLE?

Acceptance also means figuring out how to manage difficult people in our lives. You know who I'm talking about—we all have one or two or three. (Therapist protip: if it's more than three, maybe *you* should talk to someone. Just sayin'!)

Clients often come to therapy because they are dealing with difficult people in their lives—people who cause much unhappiness. One of my favorite memes is "I'm in therapy to deal with people who should be in therapy." Partially true! But prickly people create pathology in people's lives. I've seen clients who can't sleep, don't eat, and can't function at work because of how someone affects them. Toxic people bring that vibe wherever they go. Acceptance might look like acknowledging that the situation or person won't ever change and that it is unhealthy for you to be involved. In this case, you can release them and end the relationship, hopefully in a peaceful way. However, as much as we would want to end some difficult relationships, we can't. This is often true for certain work or family relationships.

I am sure you have heard "You can't change other people; you can only change yourself." This is true, to an extent. Those of you who are married know how true this can be. (I think I just heard an *Amen* from a twenty-year married person somewhere as I type this.) But we also should not underestimate the value of productive conversations and working on issues together. It's always worth trying to clarify feelings and listening. Many conflicts arise simply because we misunderstand each other and never have the opportunity to clarify.

Yet we do have to accept certain things in other people—traits that we have no power to change no matter how much we've tried. One way we can release some of those stressful emotions is to reframe the situation or see it from another perspective. One technique that can help is looking at your difficult relationship or any challenging situation from a random outsider's perspective. How would your dentist or hairdresser or mail carrier describe this situation? That might sound ridiculous, but hear me out: trying to see your difficult situation from the perspective of a random person in your life will help you simply describe the facts and remove yourself, your judgments, and your emotions from it. The research says that when we are stuck in our own rigid perspective, it is harder to practice acceptance, so seeing it from multiple angles can be helpful.

If I were to do this exercise right now, I might try taking the perspective of my hairdresser and watch myself through her eyes. I might say about myself, "I see a woman who is pretty stressed out by writing a book that's due in a few weeks. She hasn't slept much, so she probably needs to get to bed earlier. People seem annoying to her right now because she's stressed. But they are only trying to help. (Oh, and she really needs to do something with those split ends too.)"

Shifting perspective is important in helping us accept the actions of difficult people. There is usually a story behind why that person is difficult in the first place. Everyone has a story.

Maybe it's not a recent one, but an event, person, or entire childhood could have played a role in whatever annoying trait you are seeing in a person today. I often ask, "What happened to this person that makes them think that it is OK to act like this?" Perhaps if you knew, it would be easier to extend some grace.

As a therapist, I can assure you that what you see now in difficult people usually is years in the making. More often than not, it's not about you. I have also come to realize people are usually doing the best they can in any given moment based on what they have been given and how their experiences have shaped them. No, sometimes their best is not enough. But realizing that they have a story helps me give grace. But if grace is too difficult to extend—and sometimes it can be—maybe we can start by practicing acceptance.

TURNING THE KEY

- Naming emotions helps our brain sort them out and process them. This first step can help us calm down. We first must accept the emotions that accompany the situation we are trying to accept. Recognize when you are experiencing a distressing emotion and name it. Is it stress, anxiety, sadness, loneliness, or anger? Think about what specific situation may have triggered it.

- Where in your body do you feel that emotion? Perhaps you feel a heaviness in your chest or tension in your shoulders or a pit in your stomach.

- What does that emotion feel like in your body? Does it feel tight? Or painful? Or burning?

- Take a few deep breaths, and allow yourself to feel the emotion.

- Inhale for four counts. Hold it.

- Gently smile, and tell yourself it is OK to feel whatever you are feeling. Then let go and exhale, long and slow, for six counts.

CHAPTER 8

Self-Compassion

Think of someone you love. I mean really *love*. The person who could call you at 3 a.m., and you wouldn't think they were being inconsiderate. The person whose name shows up on your caller ID, and nine times out of ten, you answer the phone without a hint of resentment. *That* person. You might have only a handful of those people or maybe even just one, and that's OK. A few faces come to mind? Good. Hold on to one of them for now, and we'll come back to them.

In this chapter, we will look at self-compassion. Self-compassion and acceptance are like sisters. They like to hang out together, and you often find them borrowing each other's clothes. They are both tough, and you don't want to mess with them. But they have big, soft hearts. You know they are tight too because you've seen how they call each other every day, especially when the hard stuff hits.

You may have heard the saying "You can't really love someone until you love yourself." I can see what the aphorism is alluding to: if we are constantly looking for validation for our own worthiness, we may not truly be able to love another person unconditionally. Yet although that adage exudes an air of wisdom, I have worked with many a client who has been very good at loving other people yet had tremendous difficulty loving themselves. I will say this: it is nearly impossible to find contentment if we are constantly acting as our own adversary.

We have to come to terms with all of ourselves—the good, the fearful, the embarrassing, and the straight-up nasty—in a loving, gentle, and balanced way. We often don't know how to do this for ourselves. Many of us have a detailed, critical monologue running on replay. We may not even be aware of how negative it sounds. That's because we are so used to it, we don't even notice it. It has gotten quite comfortable.

I asked one of my clients, Mariela, to write down the things that she says to herself over the course of a day. She, like many women, struggled with self-esteem. We knew that this particular issue for her went back to middle school. I had forgotten how tumultuous those years could be until my own daughter started middle school. Many of you moms of girls just let out a deep sigh because you *know* what I'm talking about.

We often internalize these critical voices so deeply that they become the voices of *our own* monologues. I see this especially when a client grew up with critical parents or a negative family member. Research confirms that kids who grew up with critical caregivers often become highly critical toward themselves in adulthood. I asked Mariela to write down the things she tells herself over the course of a day. When she returned a week later, she told me she was utterly shocked. She hadn't realized how negative her self-talk had become and how often she found herself thinking these thoughts. Among them were *You are so ugly, You shouldn't have said that, They probably think you are stupid now, You've gained so much weight,* and *You should exercise more instead of watching Netflix.* Her thoughts were cruel and blunt, without even a trace of compassion.

"Would you talk that way to your friends if they were going through something similar?" I asked.

"Of course not!" she replied, horrified by the thought.

"I'm glad to hear that—because if you did, they probably wouldn't hang out with you," I went on. "So if your friend found herself in those same situations and you saw her struggling, what would you say to her?"

"Well . . . I guess I would say that she looked great," she said. "That everyone gains weight sometimes, and that it's frustrating, but she will lose it. I would tell her to be patient with herself. That no one is thinking about what she said at work and that she probably is her own worst critic."

"Wow." I paused for dramatic effect. "Amazing how fast you had the right words for your friend!" I paused again, hoping that would sink in, and then gently suggested, "Maybe it would be easier to hang out with yourself if you treated yourself with the same kindness."

Isn't that the truth? Most of us know exactly what we would say to a good friend or what a good friend would say to us. Think of the friend I asked you to think about at the beginning of the chapter. We know what that wise, loving person in our lives would say to *us* if we went to them. When we treat ourselves as worthy, lovable, human, and, yes, fallible, *that* is practicing self-compassion.

Compassion literally means "to suffer with." In Latin, *com* means "with" or "together" and *passion* means "to suffer." At the heart of self-compassion, then, is the idea that we can *suffer with ourselves*. We can actually be there *for* ourselves in our own pain. We can have our own back in those times we find we are alone, searching for strength and comfort. If we learn how to practice self-compassion, we don't always have to look far for support.

Mindfulness is a large part of self-compassion. We need to be aware of our own feelings of discomfort or distress in order to be present in them and accepting of them. If we don't stop to recognize our feelings, we can easily be consumed by their intensity. Mindfulness helps us sort them out in some way rather than be completely overwhelmed by them.

When I was in labor, I knew I could be swept away not only by the pain but by my emotional distress in response to the pain. I had to try to separate the two. Instead, if I tracked the length of the contractions, focused on breathing through the pain, and paid attention to how the pain actually felt physically and its location, I was able to stay more centered and get through it. Mindfulness can serve as an anchor, stabilizing us during these powerful waves of emotion.

Mindfulness can also cultivate an awareness that suffering is a shared human experience. When we go through something hard, we often feel like it is only happening to us. That creates a sense of loneliness and isolation that intensifies pain. Rather than thinking that everyone else is doing fine, we recognize that the feelings we are having are emotions that everyone experiences at some point in some way. Everyone suffers, and maybe our suffering is less unique or isolated than we think. For example, perhaps it won't feel *as* bad when we get laid off from our job if we can remember others who have been laid off as well. Perhaps we think of others who are suffering in a situation that may be harder to resolve than our own, like a scary diagnosis or a relationship issue. When we do this, we are reminded we are not the only ones in pain and therefore not alone.

Kristin Neff, author of *Fierce Self-Compassion* and the leading voice on self-compassion, defines three components of self-compassion: mindfulness, connectedness, and self-kindness. Mindfulness directs us to stay present and aware of what we are feeling, connectedness reminds us that we all suffer and are not alone, and self-kindness encourages us to treat ourselves with the kindness we extend to others. She describes these as the three legs of a stool. I like that analogy because it makes me think of self-compassion as a solid support that we can rest on when things get difficult. We can depend on these practices of self-compassion to steady us in times when we need strength.

SELF-ESTEEM VERSUS SELF-COMPASSION

In light of our conversation on the need for validation, I think you will be very interested in the difference between self-compassion and self-esteem. Both serve a similar purpose, but the differences are quite amazing. In the past decade, there has been a serious push for people to improve their self-esteem. As much as social media makes us question our sense of worth and validity, it also serves as the ultimate venue for over-the-top, almost disingenuous self-confidence. Phrases such as "You do you, boo" and "I am enough" permeate our feeds constantly.

We know from the research that this self-esteem movement has been linked to an epidemic of narcissism in college students. But it's not just college students who are affected by it.

The problem with self-esteem as we know it today is that it is almost solely based on comparison and achievement. We derive our sense of worth by looking at others and evaluating how we are doing in comparison to them. If we are doing better than someone else (downward social comparison), our self-esteem increases. If we compare ourselves to someone who appears to be sailing through life (upward social comparison), then our self-esteem takes a hit. Both types of comparison can be useful—to an extent. Being mindful of those who are not thriving in the ways you are can inspire a sense of gratitude: "I'm grateful that I have the opportunities I do today." Looking at those who are doing better emotionally or relationally in some other way can also inspire a stronger work ethic: "I want to work harder to get to that level." When our sense of self and worthiness *depends* on these comparisons, however, they can be extremely dangerous.

I don't know about you, but sometimes I read those almost toxic self-esteem declarations and think, *But I know I'm not enough all the time. I disappoint and fail and drop the ball time and again. "You do you"? Does that mean I ignore what everyone else wants and that whatever I want goes?* These statements always trigger a type of cognitive dissonance—that unsettled feeling that results from internal conflict about attitudes, beliefs, or behaviors. To me, they are thinly veiled *should* statements telling me how I need to feel. If I *don't* feel this way, then what? Am I less of a confident woman? Will I be less successful? *Do I not have healthy self-esteem?*

These statements can be confusing and even harmful. I have seen people minimize the impact of their actions on others and their families to pursue what they want at all costs. I have seen a false sense of self-esteem that actually masks deep insecurity—and, more often than not, a fear of failure. Simplistic declarations about self-esteem can become a well-constructed defense mechanism. If I don't see what needs to be seen in myself—if I can cover it with these bold affirmations—then I don't need to address it and, better yet, I won't fail.

Remember the beach ball analogy—that which we resist persists? We can push those fears under the surface for a time, but they will emerge at some point in some way. That's not to say that we live our lives doing what everyone else wants. Rather, we need the discernment that comes from authentically looking at all aspects of ourselves, which these "You do you!" statements often do not encourage. Genuine self-esteem is the ability to look at all parts of ourselves and accept them wholeheartedly and with compassion. Can we be confident enough to admit we fail and acknowledge our mistakes—and *still* believe we are inherently worthy? Can we work to change the parts of us that hold us back rather than deflect and deny them?

In order for us to feel at peace and to find calm, our sense of worthiness cannot be based on performance, achievement, or comparison. Sure, we can be proud of our accomplishments. However, it's important to recognize that success will naturally fluctuate throughout the course of our lives. And if our worthiness depends on it, we will constantly seek to one-up, produce more than, and outperform someone else as a measure of it.

Practicing self-compassion validates our sense of self simply by reminding us that we are human beings worthy of love, kindness, and compassion. Our worth is not based on performance or achievement, so we can fail and still feel worthy. We can stop producing and still feel worthy. We are not machines; we are humans: living, breathing beings with a spirit-filled soul. We are worth far more than we realize.

Self-compassion is more stable than self-esteem because it is not contingent on our success at work, at home, with our families, or in our social circles. Self-compassion acknowledges and *expects* failure because it is part of *all* our human experiences. It seems almost paradoxical that by acknowledging failure and inadequacy, we actually become more self-assured and at peace. Yet this is exactly what happens. And we have more than three thousand studies to confirm just how well it works.

THE INCREDIBLE BENEFITS OF SELF-COMPASSION

In a moment, you will learn the astounding benefits that come from a self-compassion practice. But first, let's consider why people may not be completely sold on self-compassion.

People often think, *If I just accept that I'm going to fail, then I will just be a failure and won't try harder to overcome obstacles or challenges. I won't hold myself accountable, and I won't grow.* We think accepting our weaknesses means lowering our standards and settling for less.

Our culture teaches us that the path to growth and change is through self-criticism. Beat yourself up if you fail so you will be less likely to do it again. To some extent, criticizing yourself works. Many accomplished people criticize and punish themselves until they achieve high levels of success. The problem is that they are motivated by fear: fear of failure, fear of appearing less than. They feel like they constantly need to prove their worthiness through new success and their worth is only as good as their output. This perpetual striving, however, is exhausting. Our high school students, who are pushed to their limits to achieve, will tell you they are exhausted. Many adults rarely stop to enjoy the success they've worked for. If there is another level of success to attain, they strive to keep up to sustain these feelings of worthiness. When your sense of worthiness is fueled by criticism, there is potential for great anxiety, especially performance anxiety. And when we are afraid to fail, we tend to procrastinate even more, because fear creates very real resistance to doing that thing.

Self-compassion eliminates the internal resistance we experience when we get hung up on our mistakes. When people make mistakes, they often find it hard to move on and get to their goals, and they get stuck. Self-compassion automatically eliminates *should* statements. Without this type of internal resistance, it becomes easier to pick ourselves up and move on after a setback. I know, easier said than done! Hang on for a minute and we'll get there. First, though, I want you to know how this practice of self-compassion can change your life.

We know from numerous studies that people who practice self-compassion achieve high levels of success. Instead of being motivated by fear, they are motivated by their love for themselves and by a genuine desire to do well. They try hard because they are in sync with what they *want* rather than what our culture tells them they *need*. Studies have proven that self-compassion also results in the following:

- greater levels of happiness, optimism, and life satisfaction

- greater body appreciation, perceived competence, and motivation

- lower levels of depression, anxiety, rumination, body shame, and fear of failure

- lower incidences of eating disorders, psychosis, bipolar disorders, and PTSD

- better immune response and lower levels of stress

- increased empathy toward others

- increased grit (our ability to stick to something)

- greater motivation to change and self-improve

- greater self-worth and lower levels of narcissism

I don't want to overload you with all the details of the research, but if you are into that kind of thing, the studies are listed in the notes section at the back of the book. But let's look in more depth at the link between stress and self-compassion, because this is something that moves us away from contentment on a daily basis.

STRESS AND SELF-COMPASSION

Stress affects our ability to be compassionate to both ourselves and others—which is unfortunate because stressful times are when we need self-compassion the most! I'm sure you know how hard it is to be kind to yourself when you are upset. What you might not know is that things are happening neurobiologically that also make compassion difficult when stress hits.

Oxytocin is the hormone that promotes bonding, togetherness, and closeness. We usually see it play an active role in childbirth and breastfeeding. Oxytocin also affects our ability to be empathic. One study revealed that when oxytocin was sprayed into the nose of a subject, that person demonstrated more generosity toward others, increased gazing into the eyes of another, greater empathic concern, and a better ability to read emotional states by facial expressions (an important skill in recognizing when empathy is needed). For both males and females, empathy increased with the presence of oxytocin. Interestingly enough, empathy in males increased to the baseline level of empathy found in women. Women may be naturally inclined to give empathy to others, but we definitely need reminders to extend it to ourselves.

The problem with stress is that it triggers the production of cortisol, our main stress hormone. When we are continually stressed, we produce high levels of cortisol. Like a circuit breaker designed to shut off when there's a surge or overload, excessive amounts of cortisol will eventually shut down the HPA (hypothalamic-pituitary-adrenal) axis, which produces cortisol. But when the HPA axis shuts down, other important hormones, including oxytocin, also decrease. Less oxytocin may be one of the reasons it's harder to be compassionate to ourselves or others when we are stressed. When the axis becomes suppressed, the body does not regulate stress and energy levels effectively, which impacts our immune function too. Symptoms of this HPA axis dysregulation include anxiety, depression, fatigue, and lowered immunity. Ironically, chronic stress shuts down the very system we need for a healthy stress response.

A practice of self-compassion, however, enables us to tolerate difficult emotions such as grief, despair, anxiety, anger, and shame. That thereby reduces stress and helps regulate the stress response and improve our overall immune response too. Because we are truly integrated beings, self-compassion not only improves our emotional well-being; it has a *significant* impact on our physical health too.

WHAT DOES EVERYDAY SELF-COMPASSION LOOK LIKE?

From the time he was a toddler, my son Samuel has been hard on himself. He hated to lose any sort of game. Red faced and tearful, he would run away, hide, and refuse to talk about it. Losing is less of an issue for him now that he is an adolescent, yet I have seen that same frustration appear when he can't figure something out easily, whether it be a skill in soccer or a new song on the guitar. As a cognitive therapist, I can see the thoughts flying around in his head and that momentary self-loathing become clearly visible on his face. This is exactly the type of situation that necessitates self-compassion.

Once Samuel was invited to a guitar clinic to learn to develop his skills with other students who were several years older than he was. Right away he started asking me questions like, "How long has everyone been playing?" and "How old are the kids who will be there?" I knew he was already assessing how he would feel if he wasn't as good as the other guitarists. This is a great example of the process of finding our self-esteem through comparison. He was mentally sizing people up to see where he fit in. At the time, Samuel was only twelve and likely to be the youngest player there, and he had only been playing for a little over a year. All things considered, he was pretty good for a beginner. Yet I know my son and knew this situation had the potential to unleash the beast if it didn't go well.

So I told him we had to have a talk. Kids generally don't love when a parent says that. When that parent is a therapist, it's ten times worse. I told him that when he got there, if he found that the songs were too hard and that he wasn't getting them right away, I wanted him to do a few things. "If you feel frustrated when you aren't getting the notes right away, tell yourself that it's OK to feel frustrated," I told him. "Notice where you feel the frustration, whether it's a tightness in your chest or a faster heartbeat. Take a few, slow deep breaths to calm down, and let that frustration go. You will play better if you are calmer. Remind yourself that you have only been playing for a year and are pretty good, right?" He agreed. "Remind yourself that everyone struggles at the beginning. Remember that you are the youngest one there and that with practice, you will figure it out."

This was the first time I had walked my son through how to be self-compassionate in a setting that I knew could be challenging to him. First, I started with mindfulness: being present in the feeling, acknowledging it, and accepting it. Once he was aware of the feeling, he could try to let it go through relaxation techniques, such as deep breathing (more on that later).

I then offered him basic thought replacement, which is a tenet of cognitive therapy. Thought replacement means being ready with go-to self-compassionate thoughts to replace negative ones that pop up. If he focused on "I'm pretty good for only playing for a year," that thought might even prevent negative thoughts from showing up. Lastly, I connected him to the universal experience of being a beginner so that he would know he was not alone in that frustration and that what he was feeling was normal for someone starting something new. That way it would no longer be his struggle alone; it would be one shared by many novice players.

When he got home after the guitar clinic, I heard loud footsteps running up the stairs. I could tell by the excitement in his eyes that it had gone well. "Everyone was older, and some people were really good, and I did OK," he said. "Some parts were hard, but I said the things that you told me to . . . they helped. It was fun, and I'll go again."

It is so much better for our kids to inherit a self-compassionate voice rather than a critical one. Sometimes we have to show them how to do this explicitly by giving them—and ourselves—the words. The research proves that when we practice self-compassion, we can be more fully present, develop some grit, and demonstrate a greater willingness to keep going. I saw that even in a twelve-year-old that day.

YOU ARE NOT WHAT YOU FEEL

Self-compassion might look different for you than it did for Samuel. For some of my male clients, self-compassion includes remembering that it's healthy to feel certain emotions despite the fact that they have been socialized not to. It's learning to talk about them with someone they trust so they don't internalize them, which leads to more stress and serious health issues. I'm amazed at how infrequent it is for men to talk to other men about important things! I can't count how many times my husband has returned home from seeing friends who are going through something hard—a divorce, unemployment, illness—and when I ask, "Did you talk about that?" the answer is no! Now that you understand the connection between stress and a healthy immune response, you can see why vulnerability can keep us physically and emotionally healthy. We have to encourage more of this in our men and boys.

For my clients who are new moms, self-compassion might be reminding themselves that they aren't a terrible mother if they don't love every moment with their baby who isn't sleeping or their two-year-old who is constantly throwing tantrums. It's being present in their own sadness, frustration, and guilt. It's letting go of the guilt and accepting that it's normal to feel this way during a time that's "supposed to be" joyful.

(Be warned: "supposed to be" is a *should* statement in disguise.)

For me these days, self-compassion means remembering that my body has been the first home to four children. It's remembering the time they embraced me in a group hug while I was exercising and told me, "We don't want a skinny mama; we love our squishy, soft mama." It's knowing that no matter how *I* think I look, this body will always look like home and love and safety to them, just the way it is.

Self-compassion is reassuring ourselves that going through this hard thing is normal, that others have experienced it, and that we are not alone. It is recognizing that feelings are not forever and that they will pass. You are not how you feel. Just because you feel like a terrible person doesn't make you one. Feelings often don't accurately describe one's reality but rather are reactions to whatever is happening in the present moment.

I often tell my clients, "You can't help how you feel, because feelings come and go, but you can choose how to respond to them." Self-compassion is always a good choice.

One of the most important things you can do during tough times is ask yourself, *What do I need right now?* Much like we would ask a friend who is suffering. When we ask that question, we often realize that we can do things to soothe our own pain. Sometimes that involves acts of self-care: taking a walk, meditating, calling a friend, exercising. Sometimes we have to challenge the thoughts we are having, as I did with my son. Sometimes it means simply resting.

DBT teaches what are called *distress tolerance skills*. These are skills that help us tolerate the hard emotions and situations that trigger stress. One of the ones I have used the most with clients is the five-senses technique. You can engage your senses of sight, sound, touch, smell, and taste to feel calmer. Find an object or scene that is soothing to look at (sight), such as a peaceful lake, a bouquet of flowers, or a beautiful painting. Smelling a fragrant candle (smell); wrapping yourself in a soft blanket or stroking a lovable puppy (touch); listening to peaceful, inspiring music (sound); or drinking a warm cup of coffee (taste) all provide comfort when we feel dysregulated. You can even do this exercise using your imagination by visualizing these things, and it is just as effective. In fact, that's the only way I teach it to clients in my office.

Touch is a powerful soothing sense. If you are taking deep breaths, try placing your hands on your heart to center yourself. Giving yourself a firm hug exerts a stabilizing pressure that can settle frazzled nerves. Even rocking, much like we do with children, can quiet the anxious adult. Using our senses, we actually have great power to soothe ourselves compassionately during moments of intense emotion.

Like any new skill, self-compassion takes time and practice. Because my training is in cognitive therapy, I believe that *our thoughts are everything*. Our thoughts are always a good place to start. Just know this: changing your thoughts and speaking to yourself kindly might not always feel comfortable or genuine. I tell my clients that learning to be compassionate with yourself is a bit like wearing your favorite jeans right out of the dryer. They are tight and uncomfortable at first (at least mine are), and they almost don't feel like they belong to you. But the longer you wear them around, the more you will feel at home in them. Funny, though, how comfortable the negative, self-critical thoughts feel. They might not make us feel good, but they sure are comfortable, and we tend to wear them well.

Again, start with one small change and then move on to another. Little by little, with consistency and the power of neuroplasticity, those scripted, healthy responses will very much become your own. My guess is that once you feel just how comfortable self-compassion is, you will settle down, stay awhile, and hopefully never go back.

TURNING THE KEY

- Take one day and jot down the thoughts you have about yourself. Pay attention to your thoughts when you look in the mirror, when you come up against something frustrating, or when you make a mistake or fall short. Think about an area of your life where you need to practice self-compassion. When are you hard on yourself?

- Pick one of these situations and write down a kinder, more loving response, just as you would respond to a dear friend. Say it to yourself—three times. Write it on a sticky note, and put it somewhere you will see it often.

- Take a deep, slow breath as you smile. Exhale and say to yourself, "That feels much better."

CHAPTER 9

Gratitude

I don't need to tell you that 2020 was the year of the unexpected. A few weeks into the year, we were met with the biggest shock of our lives: a global pandemic. Anxiety, depression, and paralyzing fear gripped our world as we began to navigate the uncertainties of this unwanted new normal. Yet as heart wrenching as that year proved to be—trying of our every last nerve and exhausting of every last drop of our resilience—there was one last surprise left to be uncovered.

Turns out that 2020 was our happiest year in quite a while.

It hasn't looked very good for the United States and happiness since the 1990s. According to statistics from the World Happiness Report, the last ten years have gotten consistently worse, with the United States ranking lower and lower on the reported happiness of its citizens each year. Happiness scores are based on six factors: GDP, life expectancy, generosity, social support, freedom, and corruption.

The Greater Good Science Center at the University of California (UC), Berkeley, referring to another global study on happiness, reported that the United States was ranked the eighteenth happiest country in the world in 2019. But in 2020, we jumped up four spots to fourteen. This was our best ranking in years. The World Happiness Report also confirmed the United States reported an *increase* in happiness in 2020.

How can this possibly be? During one of the most challenging years of our collective national life, how did we get *happier*?

Of course, writing about contentment, I've been thinking through this rather unusual finding. Although 2020 was the year of many things, one thing stood out for many: it truly was a year of *gratitude*.

We held our loved ones—those we could—tighter. We reached out to those we couldn't be with in person to connect, to commiserate, and to tell them we loved them. Instead of constantly being reminded of what we couldn't do, we focused on what we could. Instead of fixating on what we didn't have, we were forced to look at what we did. We collectively began to see what was truly important.

We heard about immense suffering, and we felt deeply for those losing loved ones to this deadly disease, which put our own limitations into perspective. I have never heard more people say that they were grateful for their health and their family than I did in 2020. We witnessed the heroic acts of essential workers, from doctors to grocery store clerks, putting their lives on the line every day so we could survive. And let's not forget about the delivery drivers, who gave us a sense of normalcy and offered just about the only dopamine hit we could get in those days. Never have I been so excited to see someone in my life—even if it only meant a new box of sidewalk chalk! We've seen what these folks did day in and day out forever, but this was the year we became truly grateful for them.

We played board games and did movie nights. We took long nature walks and had evening chats around a fire pit. Simple pleasures. Yes, anxiety was at an all-time high in April 2020, as the pandemic deepened. But as we approached the summer months, we began to appreciate this new, simpler way of life: more time, less rush, better weather, and finally seeing friends and family safely at a distance.

And FOMO was almost nonexistent. No one was taking glamorous vacations, so there were no photos of the crystal-clear Caribbean Sea to envy. There were no parties to be excluded from; no golf outings you weren't invited to; no women in fabulous, sparkly outfits and designer heels to envy. In some ways, the playing field was leveled. We looked at posts of how people set up their kids' classroom space at home or how families gathered around the dinner table for the first time in years.

I would never claim we were consistently "happy" that year. I don't want to minimize the extreme stressors that affected so many, especially those who lost loved ones to the virus and those who lost jobs and houses and apartments due to the pandemic. Therapists witnessed anxiety and depression skyrocket, and emergency rooms across the country were filled with young people contemplating suicide or recovering from failed attempts. This was the year of the both/and: both peace and pain. The duality of the human experience—that we can feel both pain and joy at the same time—had never been so collectively clear. It became our new, unfamiliar normal.

I do, however, think we experienced something far more profound than happiness. Perhaps calm can be found in the midst of chaos. Perhaps contentment and struggle are not mutually exclusive. Because according to the reports, we did find contentment, and we realized we didn't need all that we'd thought we needed to be happy. And in 2020, we found as many ways as possible to express how grateful we were for what we did have.

Gratitude is powerful.

I was raised in a family that believes every good thing in life is a gift. I believe that I am no more deserving of these gifts than any other human, yet many have been given to me. Gratitude comes from a place deep within my faith, and it has been passed down from generation to generation.

Even though I have always been a grateful person, two decades ago, I kind of lumped gratitude practices in with meditation, yoga, and green juice in some earth-loving, tree-hugging category that I just could not get into. I knew gratitude supposedly made you feel good, but did it make that much of a difference in the way in which we experience life? Was it worth my time to actually commit to a regular practice?

As I began researching more and learning more, however, the evidence was compelling. Seeing the brain science that supported practices of gratitude, I began to incorporate it not just into my own life but into my clinical practice. What I now know is that gratitude is not only *one* of the eight keys to contentment; it might be *the* key.

THE PRACTICE OF GRATITUDE

I met Lucian on my daughter Carolina's first day of preschool. With big brown eyes, boundless energy, and a heart-melting smile that will probably get him out of any trouble during middle school, Lucian is *that* kid. Carolina, who was three at the time, quickly scoped him out as one of her BFFs for the next two years. His ability to withstand the drama of this little curly-haired queen, in and of itself, says volumes about his perseverance.

What you would never know simply by looking at him is that Lucian spent the first three months of his life in the new-born intensive care unit (NICU). He knows the story of how he didn't come home with his mom and how his dad and older brother, Logan, who was two at the time, would come to the window to see him. He knows he weighed only a little more than three pounds, and he knows that people at the hospital helped him get healthy. The reason he knows this is because he celebrates them every year on his birthday.

For the past seven years, Lucian has celebrated each birthday with a visit to the doctors and nurses in the NICU at Greenwich Hospital. It's a family affair, in which he, Logan, and their parents, Jason and Danielle, visit the unit, arms laden with baked goods, sandwiches, gift cards, and rainbow-sprinkled cupcakes. It is a day that the family looks forward to and one that the staff adores. Danielle recounts that when Lucian was three years old, he did not understand the need for this visit . . . until he arrived, that is. But as the staff embraced him joyfully, she noticed tears well up in his eyes. Danielle remembered, "Those were not of sadness; those were tears of joy." Something within this miraculous boy recognized that he was a part of something larger, and he responded innocently and emotionally. This gratitude tradition is now written into their yearly calendar.

Danielle and Jason remember how fortunate they were to leave the NICU with a baby, and they think about how many parents of premature or ill infants do not. She says about their annual gratitude tradition, "It never feels like an obligation. It is a privilege to be there, and it helps us hold on to that feeling of gratitude for all that was given to us." Their visits also inspire and encourage the parents on the floor who feel the sadness and fear of having a child in the NICU. "I think it gives them hope to see the possibilities."

I have told this story several times, and even writing about it still brings tears to my eyes. It is a beautiful example of the power of gratitude that affects not only the recipients but those involved in the expression. Lucian and his brother are growing up understanding the importance of gratitude, which has become a *normal part of their life*. If only we were all taught such rituals of gratitude.

What if bringing joy to others through gratitude just became a normal part of life? What if that was a measure of success too? What if we were taught that gratitude was as important as an A on a test or a winning goal? How much healthier would we and our children be?

MORE THAN A FEELING

More than twelve years of research and eleven thousand pieces of data led social scientist and author Brené Brown to believe that the practice of gratitude enables one to live a "wholehearted life." Even more so than just feeling thankful every so often, *practicing* gratitude invites joy into our lives. Gratitude is more than just a feeling; it is a *choice* we make. Brown recalls not one interview in which a person who described themselves as "joyful" did not actively practice gratitude. As you can see from Lucian's story, a gratitude ritual has the power to affect far more than oneself; it invites joy, especially when it involves connection.

According to the ancient Roman scholar and statesman Cicero, gratitude is the "greatest virtue" or the "mother of all virtues." Choosing gratitude naturally leads to developing other positive qualities, such as resilience, patience, empathy, and humility. Gratitude keeps us focused on the present. We don't get drawn into the fears of the future when we are thinking of what we are thankful for today. In that way, gratitude is also a type of mindfulness that takes us by the hand and guides us to the doorway of contentment. Once we have experienced this comfortable, familiar place, we will long to return. And when you are grateful, things are happening in your brain to ensure you do just that.

ADDICTED TO GRATITUDE?

There is a biological basis for the connection between gratitude and happiness. You often cannot have one without the other. It is difficult to deny the validity of that statement when looking at the neuroscience that supports it. Research out of UC Berkeley and published in the *Wharton Healthcare Quarterly* and the *Wall Street Journal* describes what the brain looks like "on gratitude." Different types of gratitude practices impact different areas of the brain, yet all of them stimulate a release of beneficial, mood-elevating neurochemicals. And who doesn't need more of *those*?

By now you know all about dopamine and the natural high it can give you, especially when you are experiencing something new or novel. We often hear about dopamine in relation to addictive behaviors. According to research, expressing gratitude or showing gratitude to someone else also bathes the brain in dopamine, resulting in that natural high. As you might recall from an earlier chapter, the brain remembers rewards and then hardwires the message: repeat the behavior that produced it. So yes, when practiced consistently, gratitude can become addictive.

Dopamine is also linked to the following:

- increased social behavior or desire to connect with others

- increased intrinsic motivation to accomplish a goal

- increased productivity

You can see why gratitude could be incredibly valuable in schools and in the workplace. The benefits of expressing gratitude over a period of time clearly outweigh that simple moment of thankfulness. I'll get into that in just a bit.

Serotonin, also known as our "happy molecule" and the focus of many antidepressants, is released by practicing gratitude specifically through writing. We have seen that serotonin increases in response to gratitude journaling, or writing down what we are thankful for. Serotonin naturally enhances our mood, increases our willpower, and increases motivation. This makes sense, right? When we feel happier, we feel like doing more of those things that benefit us and have a positive effect on our well-being.

Although some of my clients are wary of medication for anxiety and depression, I'm a big fan of it when needed. One of my favorite lines written by Glennon Doyle is "Jesus loves me, this I know. For He gave me Lexapro." Amen to that, sister. I have seen people literally get their lives back in a matter of weeks with the *right medication*. I understand why people are averse to it due to sensitivities and side effects. It is a trial-and-error process to find the right medications. Some clients are resistant to medication because they feel it will inherently alter who they are. However, when we are anxious or depressed, we already don't feel like ourselves.

Having said that, I do think that many of us don't have to be on meds forever. Engaging in practices that naturally stimulate the release of these same mood-elevating neurochemicals can enhance the effects of medications, help us come off them at some point, and even prevent the need for them in many cases. When my patients are coming off meds, I make sure we have a plan in place that includes a gratitude practice.

So why should we engage in these behaviors regularly? I have mentioned neuroplasticity a few times now, and this characteristic of our brain remains so important in helping us understand contentment. The more regularly we engage in gratitude practices, the more we activate these neural circuits, which send signals to the brain that flag these activities as important. The brain then begins to create more myelinated neurons, structures to help the message travel faster and strengthen this pathway. At the same time, the brain is fantastic at conserving neural energy, so it begins to degrade pathways that we don't use as much or at all. So if gratitude helps you begin to appreciate more and complain less, those complaining pathways will eventually degrade. If we don't use them, we don't need them. More neural pathways that support the release of dopamine and serotonin mean a generally happier and more contented state. All this emerges from simple and frequent acts of gratitude. Remember, what we think about grows stronger.

So you can literally change the structure of your brain so that it becomes more efficient at producing neurochemicals that *promote* happiness. Essentially, you can hardwire your brain for contentment. The key is time and consistency—although perhaps less time than you would think. One study set out to determine what effect writing a gratitude letter would have on people experiencing anxiety and depression. A group of three hundred adults who had just starting regular counseling were separated into three groups. The first group was instructed to write one gratitude letter per week for three weeks. They could write about what they were thankful for or a note of thanks, and they were not required to send the letter to someone unless they chose to. The second group was asked to write out their deep thoughts and feelings about a negative experience, and the third group was asked to do nothing more than attend the counseling sessions.

Four weeks after the study was completed, the group that wrote the letters reported significantly better mental health than the other two groups. *Twelve* weeks later, individuals in that same group continued to thrive; MRIs of their brains showed even stronger activity in the medial prefrontal cortex, the area important for mood regulation. You should know that only 23 percent of that group actually *sent* the letters, but the results were consistent for all of them, regardless of whether they mailed their letters or not.

The act of simply writing about positive experiences and emotions shifts the brain away from toxic negative thoughts and distressing feelings. The results also suggest that gratitude practices not only have benefits in the moment; greater benefits to mood and well-being actually accrue over time.

GRATITUDE: IT DOES A BODY GOOD

Studies have also revealed that in addition to increasing emotional and psychological well-being, a regular practice of gratitude has physical health benefits.

- The Greater Good Science Center details studies that correlate those who kept gratitude journals for two weeks with improved health such as fewer headaches, less congestion, and fewer sore throats, coughs, chest pains, and stomachaches.

- The same study reported those who took the extra step to express gratitude to someone sustained these health benefits for several weeks after the study had ended.

- Grateful cardiac patients reported better sleep, less fatigue, and lower levels of inflammation. Patients with heart failure who kept gratitude journals for eight weeks had reduced signs of inflammation afterward.

- Several studies also suggest that gratitude can improve the quality of sleep even in those with sleep disorders.

A word to the wise: keep your gratitude practices simple. Short and sweet is just as effective as long and complicated in experiencing the benefits of gratitude. Two easy ways you can begin are by journaling and by expressing gratitude.

GRATITUDE JOURNALING

Gratitude journals now come in all shapes, sizes, and methods. I'm sure some of you are already exhausted by thinking about writing *every day*. But there are ways to accomplish this task and enjoy the benefits of journaling that can suit even those who don't care for writing. Studies reveal that it is actually more beneficial to reflect and write every *three days* rather than each day—perhaps because we have more to reflect upon.

I keep a separate journal just for gratitude. Because time is always limited, I simply bullet-point moments and events I want to remember. I do have another journal to record other life events, including the not-so-positive things that I need to process. (By the way, writing is a great way to take out emotion and process negative experiences on a paper rather than on a person. You can't write as fast as you think, so it slows thought processes down and enables you to pause and think through what you are feeling.)

I love keeping a separate journal simply for gratitude because on days when I am feeling low and need to be reminded of all that is good in my life, I can find all those reminders in one place. I know myself well: I could have had a fantastic day on Monday, but if a tough day hits midweek, I will have forgotten all those good things that happened by Friday. This way when I get in a funk, I don't have to sift through stories and countless other experiences detailed in my everything journal to find the good things I've experienced. An entire journal dedicated to positive and joyful moments, people, and things is a powerful tool for cultivating contentment. (If you are over forty-five like I am, you don't even remember what you had for dinner last night. So unless you write these beautiful things down, fuhgeddaboudit—because you will.)

Elaborating on the events you're recording—including details about the person or experience you are grateful for—is fantastic. But you can also keep it short and sweet and receive similar benefits of journaling. Using vivid descriptions, even if they're short, will help you remember the moment five years from now.

Clients often ask me this question about gratitude journals: "What do you do when you are writing about the same things every day: health, family, work, relationships?" I suggest that people try to find *specific* moments or things for which they are grateful. If we take a minute to think through our day, good or bad, even in the mess, we can find moments. I love Alice Morse's words: "Every day may not be good . . . but there is something good in every day." Truth! The apostle Paul talks in the New Testament about giving thanks not *for* all things but "*in* all things." We likely take things for granted that someone else literally dreams about. When I drag myself out of bed in the morning not wanting to exercise, I think about the mom fighting for her life in a hospital bed. When I dread meal planning for yet another week, I think about families lined up for hours at food banks. When the noise coming from my kids fighting is deafening, I think about my kids living on their own and my home being a quiet empty nest one day. These images quickly turn my negative attitude into gratitude.

What would it mean to go through your day looking for the good moments in your imperfect and often unpredictable life? For me, drinking a hot cup of coffee without having to microwave it three times—a sheer miracle in my home—is one of those moments. (I'm serious. My daughter Natalia once gave me a mug that reads, "If found in the microwave, return to Mom.") For you it might be running into an old friend at the bookstore, noticing new blossoms on the tree outside your window, closing a huge deal at work, attending an intimate dinner party, looking at a serene winter sky, or waking up to a quiet house when all the kids are sleeping. These are simple moments—often ordinary, occasionally extraordinary—and ones that evoke joy, peace, and hope. Think of them as scenes in the movie of your life: moments that you may want to remember with clarity when you look back. Collect these moments. I often think even if nothing good happens for the rest of my life, I have already collected enough of these to last me a lifetime. These moments leave an imprint of contentment and give us the assurance that surely our lives have been full.

NOTES OF GRATITUDE

I am always moved by a handwritten thank-you note. I mean, who even does that anymore? In this digital age of instant communication, I am always amazed and moved when someone takes the time to write a message in a card, look up my postal address, put a stamp on an envelope, and send it off. Seeing old-school mail on the counter immediately makes me feel more appreciated than receiving a quick text does. I have received thank-you notes for having invited a friend to dinner, for having given a talk that someone found meaningful, and for having guided a client through a difficult process. All these notes were unexpected, and I think that's part of their beauty. In this culture of impersonal, disconnected, empathy-absent communication, the connection fostered by expressions of gratitude is vital.

Every Christmas, I send the two secretaries at my children's school small gift cards to Starbucks for all the trouble I cause with questions likely answered in emails that I haven't read. Without fail, I receive a handwritten note from each of them—*before* Christmas. These notes always stand out in my mind, because it likely takes them more time to write and send those notes than it did for me to buy the very modest gift cards! Their simple yet powerful gesture leaves me humbled and thankful for *their* thoughtfulness and grateful that such kind people are a part of our lives. Thank-you notes are powerful because this type of expressed gratitude has the potential to create and perpetuate a cycle of connection, compassion, mindfulness, and even more gratitude.

The research tells us that gratitude encourages prosocial behavior—meaning it makes people feel kind, generous, and helpful. Gratitude strengthens relationships, and many social scientists believe gratitude is essential to keep any society healthy and thriving.

When we are the recipient of someone else's gratitude, we feel connected to that person. These notes have sometimes changed the tone of my *entire* day by reminding me that someone was thinking of me and was appreciative of something that I didn't think was all that noteworthy. If someone is in a good mood, she does good things, she gets things done, she enjoys her life, she feels good, and she treats those around her a little better. It's quite incredible that such a simple act can create an ongoing ripple effect of happiness: to those who give thanks, to those who receive it, and even to those who are completely unaware of it!

Not all of us are note writers, and many other expressions of gratitude can create the same cycle of positivity. A simple verbal "thank you" can affect the way in which someone views themselves, their responsibilities, and their relationship with the person expressing it. Look for as many opportunities as you can to simply say thank you. That's something we can all do fairly easily. When my daughter Sofia thanks me for making her favorite dinner (chicken nuggets . . . all day long), it changes the way I feel about the arduous task of meal planning; it makes me feel grateful to be her mom and to see the young woman she is growing up to be. When I thank my husband for taking out the garbage, he might first pass out on the kitchen floor from shock, but then he remembers to keep doing it. Clearly I don't do it enough, but receiving a thank-you can make an unpleasant task bearable because of the emotional connection it fosters. Expressions of gratitude also validate behavior and encourage more of it when the behavior is appreciated. So especially if *we* don't want to do it, we should all be thanking whoever is taking out the trash every single time! (That's a therapist/smart wife protip!)

GRATITUDE RITUALS

Gratitude rituals can be unique and customized to what works for you and your household. One important part of gratitude is acknowledging the sources outside of ourselves that have given us these good things, whether those sources are people or a higher power. My husband and I have prayed with our kids before bedtime since they were infants. We want them to learn to recognize gifts and give thanks for them as a natural part of their lives. Prayer is now their bedtime ritual, one they actually request to peacefully fall asleep. We used to play a game called "roses and thorns," in which they name the roses, or things that were fun or made them happy in their day, as well as the thorns, or the challenges. We then give thanks for the roses, recognizing they were gifts, and pray about the thorns, which helps them let them go. Not only is this an opportunity for us as their parents to learn about their day; it gives us a glimpse into their little minds and hearts (although two out of my four are taller than me now). I can see why it is easy to fall asleep after this heart-filling focus. Research confirms that those who practice gratitude rituals before bed—including people with sleep disorders—have healthier, sounder, and longer sleep than those who do not. Certainly a better alternative to NyQuil.

So can we become addicted to gratitude? I certainly hope so. At the very least, it can become so integrated into our mindset that we naturally respond from that place.

If you have ever had your coffee paid for by the person in front of you, you know what I'm talking about. If you haven't, pay for someone's coffee next time you are buying yours, and you will see in an instant what this means. This "pay it forward" response comes to those who themselves have been recipients of an act of kindness. There seems to be a universal human desire to perpetuate this cycle of kindness once one has been a beneficiary. Maybe it's the dopamine rush that comes from this unexpected event. If this is not addictive, it is at least intoxicating and something we all can get used to.

Practicing gratitude allows us to recognize and experience the greatness of what we *have* rather than be consumed by thoughts of what we lack. It is in those moments that we truly want what we already have. Gratitude is the beating heart of contentment.

TURNING THE KEY

- Find a regular time of day and take thirty seconds to think of one thing that you are grateful for. Pick a time that works for you, such as when you open your eyes in the morning, after you take your first sip of coffee, or right before your head hits the pillow.

- Visualize that one thing that you are thankful for. Stay in it for a minute, savoring the details of that moment or person. Think about who it involves or how it makes you feel. Take a slow, long deep breath. Exhale. Say to yourself, "That makes me feel [pick one]: loved, happy, peaceful, calm, grateful."

- Try to do this every day at that same time for a week. If you start to forget, set a reminder on your phone to alert you around that time. It won't take long before this becomes just a part of who you are and how you see the world—and when that happens, be grateful for that too!

CHAPTER 10

Connection

As a therapist, I have the privilege of walking with clients through some of the darkest moments of their lives. I envision these painful experiences as rooms with doors firmly shut to most people. But my clients graciously invite me in, ask me to stay awhile, and often even allow me to explore a bit.

In my fifteen years in practice, I have seen very hard things. Some unimaginable. Some seemingly unbearable.

In these times, the only thing I can offer is presence. I don't underestimate the value of presence: it is powerful and incredibly healing. As a therapist, though, I always want to offer more: insight, knowledge, strategies, tips, and techniques. I've been trained for this. Yet I find on some of those very dark days, I can't.

One time in particular, I could not even find simple words. That day was December 14, 2012.

Like me, you might remember exactly where you were when you heard the news on that clear-blue-sky December morning. Twenty first graders and six educators were violently murdered in their classrooms at Sandy Hook Elementary School in Newtown, Connecticut—twelve miles from where I lived.

The morning after the devastation, I received a call asking if I would sing at the memorial service for Dylan Hockley, one of the little boys killed that day. His parents, Ian and Nicole, had requested to hold the service at our church. They had gotten to know our pastors, who arrived at the scene that day to support the shocked and grieving families and to pray with them.

On the day of the memorial service, I watched as this young couple, standing at the podium in front of hundreds of people, spoke of their beautiful son, an energetic six-year-old who loved the color purple, the moon, and trampolines. If I could sum up strength and grace in one image, it was exactly what they embodied in that moment.

Having stayed in touch with Ian over the years, I called him up as I was writing and asked him, "How?" *How* did they go on and find moments of joy and peace, having endured the hardest thing, in my opinion, a parent could experience? What enabled them to do so? Whatever it was, it had to be powerful, and I wanted to know more about it.

His answer in one word: friends.

Ian confirmed that the grief of Dylan's death will never go away. But their connection with friends and a support system of relationships have enabled them to find meaning and purpose in the midst of the ongoing pain. "My friends call me up and reach out especially before the hard days—birthdays, anniversaries," he told me. "They always remember. They check on me constantly." Ian started running regularly with a group of friends who have become family to him. He now races alongside them as he raises money for his nonprofit organization, Dylan's Wings of Change, a community dedicated to fostering empathy and connection in young people empowered by the belief that everyone matters.

Research confirms what Ian has discovered. Although connection to other people may not be the only way to find contentment, you will be hard-pressed to find contentment without it.

THE LOVE CONNECTION

If you thought of a dating game show when you read those words, you are old enough to know from experience that relationships have great power to influence our mood and alter our entire outlook on life. (You're probably also old enough to pull a muscle just by walking too fast to the fridge. I feel you.) This is especially true for our most intimate relationships.

I have witnessed couples with strong marriages persevere when the world around them seems to be falling apart. A connected relationship serves as a protective buffer when challenges arise. On the flip side, I have seen people who have every luxury and and seemingly perfect lives suffer terribly when their relationship is struggling. Talking to them, I know that many would trade everything they have to heal that relationship, because it feels as if their world is falling apart. If you have ever had a strained relationship with a child or spouse, you know what this feels like. When love is compromised, so is our sense of well-being.

If we are talking about the relationship between connection and contentment, we have to talk about the Harvard Grant Study, which tracked 268 Harvard sophomores for more than eighty years. The class included men who would go on to careers in all walks of life, one of whom would become the boyish young president John F. Kennedy. Sixty of these men are still alive today. The study went on to include additional subjects, men from urban areas, for a total of 724 participants, and now the 2,000 children of these men are also being followed. Essentially we're talking about a ton of data gathered over the longest time a study has ever been conducted on well-being and what it takes to be happy.

You could likely guess by now that close relationships were shown to enable people to live long, happy, and healthy lives. This finding proved true in men across the board: from the privileged halls of Harvard to the underresourced city neighborhoods of America.

What you may not know is that relationships affected far more than the subjects' moods. What if I told you that regardless of your IQ, social status, or even genes, you could live a long and fulfilled life? Now, what if I told you it was *love* that made more of a difference than any of these things? It really is hard to believe, but this is exactly what this study continues to prove. What is particularly encouraging is that in this case nurture apparently wins over nature. Some of the men came from significantly dysfunctional families and life experiences. But as long as they were willing to do the work of fostering stronger connections, these men lived longer and more fulfilled lives.

Study participants' level of satisfaction with their relationships at age fifty was a better predictor of physical health at age eighty than their cholesterol levels. Those most satisfied with their relationships at age fifty were most physically healthy at age eighty. Don't miss this: the quality of your relationships in your forties and fifties is a predictor of how healthy and long your life will be. It is not merely being in an intimate relationship or having lots of friends that afford these bene-fits. Rather, cultivating genuine, secure, and healthy attachments result in well-being. So for those of you who don't feel like you have your "group," know this: we don't need many relationships in midlife, just a few deeper, meaningful ones. (Interestingly, for adolescents and the elderly, research suggests a wider social net-work is more important for well-being than deep connections.)

So how many of these friendships do you actually need in order to reap these benefits in midlife? When it comes to close relationships, researchers have determined fifteen to be the typi-cal number for humans, based on our brain's capacity to invest in close connections. This number decreases to five when we are talking about our innermost circle, which includes a romantic partner, close relatives, and besties. So really, most of us don't need many friends. The most important factor is that you feel supported and not stressed out by these relationships. Who out there needs to hear this?

Unhealthy, stressful relationships have the exact opposite effect on our physical and mental health. We see this with ado-lescents quite clearly, but it is true in adulthood too. No mat-ter how old you are, our thoughts, decisions, and self-esteem are still influenced by the types of friends we spend our time with. "Show me your friends, and I will tell you who you are" is a saying found in several cultures, from Greek to Spanish. We often become reflections of those whose company we keep—so choose wisely.

In addition, researchers also found that loneliness, com-pared to being connected in healthy relationships, is mea-surably more toxic, both mentally and physically, than smoking cigarettes or drinking alcohol. The research proves a clear link between loneliness and stress and inflammation, which may contribute to the health issues we see down the line in some people. Increased risk of heart disease, stroke, and even dementia often shows up beginning in midlife. They weren't joking when they said loneliness can kill you. We also know that the more connected you are to friends in your social circle, the less likely you are to become ill—and the faster you will recover if you do.

You don't have to come from a healthy family or past to live a beautiful, meaningful life of impact. If we invest the time to seek healing and strengthen ourselves, we all have a shot at a healthy, connected life. However, if we don't heal our own open wounds, we will continue to bleed on those who never cut us.

When we can find peace and contentment on our own, we stop holding others around us hostage when they don't give them to us. Yes, a healthy connection can facilitate healing. But if we come to the table knowing how to heal, then the relationship truly becomes a gift rather than a rehab. With the right practices and support, healing is possible. Healthy connections and therefore a life of contentment are absolutely possible *for everyone*.

HARDWIRED TO CONNECT

Two of our kids have severe food allergies. If you are the parent of a child with food allergies, you know that every outing to a restaurant can be quite an adventure. Our party of six is already a lot for any server to manage, and on top of that, I always have a ton of annoying allergy-related questions for them to answer. Really, the dream table are we.

For most of the meal, I am on high alert, constantly assessing if any of my kids are showing symptoms that signal the start of a life-threatening reaction. If we catch it, I can intervene early, hopefully before we need to whip out one of the four EpiPens that we carry. So you can imagine my concern a few nights ago when we ate at a restaurant that had just opened in town, and during the meal, my youngest started to complain of a stomachache. She climbed into my lap and sat awhile as I tried to finish my dinner, eating around her squirming hot body. This proved quite difficult, and since she didn't seem too sick, I gently moved her back into her seat. She sat by herself for a minute before she climbed back up, insisting, "My belly feels better when I sit on your lap."

Clearly being pressed up against her mama brought her emotional comfort. But what I didn't realize until recently was that being close to me may actually have brought *physical* relief from pain as well. This is just how hardwired we are for connection.

In the Harvard Grant Study, researchers discovered that people who had happy marriages in their eighties reported that their moods did not suffer even on days when they had more severe physical pain. Conversely, those who had unhappy relationships felt more emotional and physical pain. Remember when I said we are truly integrated beings? Emotional and physical pain are deeply intertwined, as are emotional and physical health.

There is a fascinating connection between physical pain and loneliness. If you have ever broken up with a significant other—or had *them* break up with you—you know this. You might remember that anguish almost physically, in your body. If you have experienced the death of a loved one, you know this very well. Scientists have discovered that emotional and physical pain are both experienced through the same neural network. Recent data even suggest that Tylenol, an over-the-counter medication we use for fevers and headaches, can be an effective way to reduce the pain of social loss or separation. Can you imagine?

Now I'm not suggesting that you run out and take Tylenol every time you are upset. Excessive Tylenol consumption is not without significant side effects. But the fact that pain medication can impact both the physical and the emotional demonstrates just how integrated the body, mind, and spirit truly are.

From our first moment of life, we are connected to another human. We can only make our entrance into this world through another human. We don't learn to do anything—walk, speak, or eat—on our own, but rather we mimic what we see. Our brains contain "mirror neurons," which do just that: reflect what we see so we can learn. They enable us to take in, process, and imitate information that helps us understand another person's emotions and behaviors. This is why babies imitate the expressions of their caregivers and know how to respond when you are smiling at them. Mirror neurons also foster our ability to empathize with each other: to feel and understand each other and therefore deepen these vital connections.

What my daughter described on that day at the restaurant— that her stomach felt better when I was holding her—has been confirmed through research. There is an analgesic effect—that is, pain relief—when two people *with a significant connection* touch each other in support. One experiment evaluated pairs where one of the two received a burn-like sensation. The other person held that person's hand, offering support. When the two participants were strangers, there was no observable effect. But when the two participants were in a romantic relationship or in some way emotionally connected to each other, the outcome proved very different. Researchers observed similar patterns of brain activity between the two. They noted activity in the right frontal lobe of the person *not* receiving the burn-like sensation, suggesting brain waves specific for *empathy*. Empathy brain waves mean the person *not* feeling the burn suffered emotionally with the person who *did*.

In fact, the more similar the brain waves or brain synchrony between the two, the less pain the person receiving the heat actually felt. This and other studies suggest that touch from someone we are connected to can improve our tolerance of physical pain and even decrease it. This may also explain why when a doctor touches a patient during treatment, the outcome of the interaction is better. When we hold our children as they receive a vaccine or hold a friend's hand for moral support, we may, literally, lessen their pain.

DO SCREEN CONNECTIONS COUNT?

Can you understand why our screen-addicted culture may be facing connection challenges? We know that screens contribute to the loneliness and disconnect we are seeing, especially among adolescents. We also have research to prove that there is a correlation between screen time and symptoms of anxiety and depression. A landmark 2018 study found that the less time people spent on social media, the less lonely and depressed they felt.

Loneliness and isolation proved to be significant issues even before the pandemic exacerbated them. The Centers for Disease

Control and Prevention (CDC) reported that even before the pandemic, more than a third of adults aged forty-five and older felt lonely. When it comes to teens and young adults, studies have shown that an astounding 40 percent of those aged sixteen to twenty-four report feeling lonely "often" or "very often." That's two out of every five people who reported that they do not feel connected to anyone. In these cases, not only is contentment compromised; overall physical and emotional health can suffer for years to come.

My patient, Peter, once told me that he was jealous of his wife because she had so many friends. He was happy for her but truly wished he had a group of friends to spend time with. As Peter shared his feelings, I could see that saying these thoughts out loud was tough for him. He looked embarrassed, and he revealed that he felt ashamed for even feeling jealous of someone he loved so deeply. Jealousy is an important emotion, as it often reveals our deepest longings and needs. I tell my clients to follow their jealousy to see where it leads. In this case, the need was for belonging. Although Peter felt incredibly happy in his marriage, a spouse cannot meet every need we have for connection. It isn't fair to place that burden—of meeting one's every emotional need—on one person, and if we do, it can run the risk of codependency.

Because of Peter's struggle with self-esteem, he had a hard time connecting. As we did the work of therapy, he realized that he didn't make much of an effort to reach out to friends because deep down, he felt that people would not want to be friends with him. He had been hurt by friends in the past, so he had a hard time being vulnerable and trusting people, and he often shut down opportunities that came his way. Loneliness can be a result of not working through some of our own stuff. You might be standing in your own way of finding what you truly long for.

Most of us recognize that our culture sends toxic messages to women regarding our value and worth and how they lie in our appearance and usefulness to other people. But men receive toxic messages too. Vulnerability, which is essential for deep, connected relationships, can be hard for men. We tell men they need to be vulnerable in relationships, but from the moment they enter the world, we also tell them, "Don't cry. Be strong. Fight hard." Men are quickly perceived as weak or incompetent on the sports fields, among friends, at work, and in intimate relationships when they show too much emotion and sensitivity. For this reason, a deep, meaningful connection in any relationship might be hard for some men; this is something I think about as I raise a son in our culture that hasn't changed very much in terms of our messaging.

Connecting can be difficult, especially given the busyness of our lives these days. When we spend our time trying to catch up on emails and texts, scrolling through multiple social media platforms, and running from one extracurricular obligation to the next, where is the time to deeply connect? This busyness—and lack of connection because of it—is the price of the "more" that we constantly seek. But like with anything important, if we don't make the time, a deeper connection with others will never magically appear.

Deeper connections are easier to make if two people share similar important values. When I am involved in antiracist work, I become fast friends with others involved. I may not have known them for long, but because we are connecting on something important to both of us, the connection is fast and deep.

Connecting to others through service is an ideal way to foster meaningful connections if you are looking to make them. But that's not all you will find when you decide to give of your time and resources.

BETTER TO GIVE THAN TO RECEIVE?

Many charitable organizations faced unprecedented challenges in 2020. Seeing an increase in unemployment and the number of families left hungry, many people donated to food banks at the end of the year instead of their usual charities. This left many nonprofits with a year-end gap that they struggled to close.

Carrie, a good friend of mine, heads one of these organizations in our area: a medical clinic that treats uninsured children, who are also often undocumented. Two days before Christmas, she was struggling to close a $20,000 gap in the budget so that the clinic could continue to provide desperately needed medical services to families. My mother and my sister, Krissy, both pediatricians, volunteer there. Thinking of children not getting health care, especially right before Christmas, weighed heavily on my heart. Hoping that other people may be moved in the same way, I offered to help raise some of the money to cover expenses.

Krissy and I posted a video on social media appealing for funds for the clinic. We called our forty-eight-hour quest Operation Christmas Miracle and asked our friends and followers to donate even five dollars. We knew it would be a true miracle if we could raise anything close to $20,000 in two days. We then planned to livestream the announcement of the total amount raised at the clinic on Christmas Eve. We expected to raise a few thousand dollars. What we did not expect was that donors from all over the country would eagerly get involved. This is the power of social media, one of those moments when screens can be used for extraordinary good. We heard stories of children running to their piggy banks and taking out their dollar bills to donate to "kids who didn't have money to pay for doctors." We saw people from all socioeconomic groups give generously. I'll tell you how it turned out in just a bit. But first let's ask this question: What moved people to give to a charity they had never even heard of?

Once again, according to our research in neuroscience, we are wired for compassion. I have always loved a definition of compassion that comes from Chris Kukk, author of *The Compassionate Achiever*. He writes that compassion is empathy *plus* action. It's being able to feel what someone is feeling and then take steps to do something about it. We see this in research on toddlers, who have a biological drive to help others without any reward, simply motivated by compassion. In fact, when we think about participating in an act of compassion, such as giving or volunteering, our pleasure and reward centers in the brain light up. According to the National Institutes of Health, the brain activity we see is very similar to what happens when we eat chocolate or have good sex. And I also know some of you are seriously thinking about volunteering now.

As we saw earlier, MRI studies have shown that when you empathize with someone else, your brain looks very similar to the brain of the person in pain. Makes sense, right? If you are imagining what it's like for that person to suffer, you are kind of "tricking" your brain into experiencing actual pain. When people are doing acts of compassion, the MRI images of their brains look very much like the brains of people who are in love.

Reward, pleasure, love: what good reasons to connect with others through service. And there's more.

Endorphins, our natural opiates, are released when we give of our time or resources to help another person. This is our brain's mild version of a morphine high—it has been appropriately named the "helper's high." Studies have also confirmed that giving through service releases the happiness trifecta: dopamine, serotonin, and oxytocin. So people are neurobiologically inclined to help others. Even the *thought* of meeting a need can trigger these neurochemicals and make us feel good.

Service is one thing that I encourage most for my clients to do if they aren't doing it in some capacity already. Anxiety and depression can be incredibly consuming. In no way do I want to minimize the seriousness of these illnesses and the need to care for oneself in the middle of them. But I have also seen that as we work through them, we can become completely self-focused on our own struggles and disconnected from the world around us. When we engage in acts of kindness or volunteering, we are empowered, by our own agency, to meet *someone else's needs*. We know these acts, in and of themselves, release happy neurochemicals. These opportunities also often help us step into gratitude for what we can do to make a difference. Patients suffering from anxiety and depression often feel powerless, so service helps them see that they are not without agency and find meaning in the process. These opportunities lend to self-compassion by seeing that others have needs and that they suffer too. It's not just us, and we are not alone. Through service, connection happens on multiple levels, each of which can bring healing.

Service might even save our own lives. A study out of the University of Buffalo and published in the *American Journal of Public Health* detailed that people who helped others lived longer because they were less likely to die when confronted with a stressful event. For those who were *not* helpers, each stressful event increased the chance of death over the next five years by 30 percent! The study made a positive correlation between helping, stress reduction, and good health. I was surprised that researchers could quantify exactly how service impacts our mortality. According to the study, when bad things happen, acts of kindness serve as a buffer to protect the giver.

For centuries, almost every philosophical and religious tradition has held the ideals of connecting with others through service and taking care of one's neighbors. Aristotle wrote about the concept of *Eudaimonia*, a Greek word meaning "happiness"—although it suggests that happiness is the result of human flourishing and the actualization of human potential. Aristotle reflected that a healthy, thriving person is one who takes pleasure when others are also thriving. Part of self-actualization happens when we help others attain that level too. Isn't that the truth? When we can be genuinely happy for others when they are flourishing—without feeling competitive, jealous, resentful, or self-pitying—we know we have found true contentment. As Aristotle noted, that is the mark of a person who is healthy and thriving themselves.

Buddhist teachings use the term *bodhisattva* to describe a person who encapsulates the qualities of compassion and altruism. Originating from ancient Sanskrit, this word describes a person who seeks enlightenment specifically for the purpose of liberating all beings from suffering. This is a word used for a noble person and clearly elevates the idea of service through compassion.

From my own Christian faith tradition come references all over the Bible about loving your neighbor as yourself. One of my favorites is found in 2 Corinthians 1:3–5. It has always given me a meaning for suffering, although I recognize we will never truly understand the whys in this life. I have always understood verse 4 as explaining that the reason we go through hard things is so we can comfort others who are also going through hard things, sharing wisdom and strength. It's as if that is purpose enough in this life: to be connected to others and to show compassion.

Despite their differences, philosophical and religious traditions around the globe agree that one of our greatest purposes involves connecting with and serving those around us. Thanks to brain science, we now know that the benefits of altruism surpass the actual act of generosity for both the giver and the receiver.

As for the medical clinic and Operation Christmas Miracle? Well, a miracle we asked for and a miracle we received. Hour by hour, we waited with anticipation, totaling donations of every size. We witnessed two hundred donors from across the country moved by compassion for kids they would never know. Most had completed their year-end giving and didn't ask for tax-deductible gift receipts; they simply gave out of a desire to be a part of a collective effort of compassion. There was no reward, nothing in it for them, just a feeling of being a part of something bigger and meaningful. One of these donors, three thousand miles away in California, even offered to match a portion of what we could raise.

In those forty-eight hours, we collected $38,000. We had been aiming for just a percentage of the $20,000 the clinic needed to make ends meet. As we livestreamed this reveal on social media, we felt the flood of emotion across the country, and we saw the happy tears of those who participated. It was a beautiful moment of connection and compassion and revealed how we can experience true contentment when we take care of one another.

Before we left for the clinic to announce the total, I sat at my desk in disbelief, tearfully moved by the generosity of people at the busiest time of the year. Sitting next to me was my daughter Sofia, writing the name of each donor on the inside of a giant card she had created for the clinic. On the front of the card, she had drawn planet earth, surrounded by people of every color holding hands. Beneath the picture read the caption, "Together We Can Walk on Water."

And so we did.

TURNING THE KEY

- Find one simple way to connect with someone at the same time each day. Send a text or an email or call a friend. You could do it as you get in your car in the morning, as you drink your second cup of coffee, or before you get ready for bed. Pair the act of connecting to something you do normally. Try to do this consistently for seven days.

- Once a week, reach out to a friend you care about but who you haven't spoken to recently. Or once a month, send a letter of encouragement to someone you know is going through a difficult time.

- Write these things into your calendar and block off time to do them.

- Reward yourself immediately after. That might be blissfully enjoying that cup of coffee or thinking of a happy memory that involved that person. Say to yourself, "That made me happy." This may feel awkward at first, but our brains listen to what our mouths speak.

- Even random acts of kindness are powerful in terms of increasing our sense of contentment. If you can, buy coffee or lunch for the person behind you in line somewhere. Let someone go in front of you in the checkout line. Their reaction may be a reward enough.

- Think about your own relationships. Do you feel connected and supported? Do you support others? What needs to change in your life to strengthen your connections? Do you have toxic relationships that need to be let go of? Are there new relationships that need to be fostered?

- Consider what you need to do to strengthen your connections.

CHAPTER 11

Present Focus

Few things stir my soul more than an autumn day in New England: crisp air; earthy, warm hues; and of course pumpkin-spice anything. By the end of the month, however, I find myself thinking that this season goes way too fast. One minute we are surrounded by breathtakingly beautiful, rich color, and in a blink, everything seems to disappear.

On a brisk fall afternoon, I walked to our mailbox as usual. I'm sure I was focused on one thing: getting back to the house so I could get one more thing done before the kids came home. I didn't pay attention to the crunch of crispy leaves beneath my feet, the bits of saffron and scarlet scattered on the mowed grass, or the smoky smell of wood burning nearby. I actually just made up those details now, because at the time, I didn't notice any of it. I don't remember any of those lovely sights and sounds and smells from that moment. Because we only remember what we pay attention to.

But I do remember opening a letter that day, one that I don't think I will ever forget. The letter welcomed our family and the class of 2025 to our local high school. Although we were nearly a year away from my oldest daughter attending high school, the district wanted us to be informed and ready. I felt a large lump form in my throat, and the letters on the page became suddenly blurry. High school? How did we get here so soon?

The year 2025 seemed so far away in December 2006, when we held our firstborn for the very first time. My mind flashed back to the swinging and rocking I did every night to get this colicky baby to sleep. Those were the days of sore legs and sleepless nights. People told me that it would get better in three months, but I wasn't sure I'd last three weeks. Now here we were fourteen years later, in disbelief—not quite sure where the time went. I wish someone could have told me to think of raising kids in thirds. By the time they are six years old, you are done with a third. By their middle school years, you've got two-thirds down with only one to go. That's it. Maybe it would have put things in perspective.

Walking back into the house, I began to think through all the times I had been busy or distracted while she and her siblings grew up right in front of me. Starting my own practice, packing and unpacking from several moves, managing the busyness of each new baby: Did I enjoy the time? Did I miss important things? Was I fully present?

An unsettled feeling washed over me. I wasn't sure I remembered enough of those earlier years of her life. But one thing I did know for sure: I was not going to miss another minute of my last third.

These days, we all miss a *lot* of things. Important things. Things that we will never get back because we just aren't paying attention. In fact, research says that our modern minds are wandering 47 percent of the time.

I believe it. This wandering of the mind—distracted living—is the reason that the fall seems to whiz by so fast for me. Our attention is constantly fractured, consumed by so many less important things that rob us of very important moments.

I want to show you how to get back your attention so you aren't ever left asking the questions I asked myself that day. Because nothing steals contentment like the feeling that we missed out on the one life we were given.

During the past decade of doing therapy, I have witnessed two things that constantly prevent people from living in the present. One is cell phones, and the other is anxiety. They are actually more related than they sound.

GET OFF YOUR PHONE

"Get off your phone": if I had a dollar every time someone in my family has said this to me, I would be writing this book from a seaside resort in Jamaica. Phones are the number-one cause of distraction for most of us. Why? Because they are usually right at our fingertips.

We've already talked about why we are drawn to social media and how that validates some of our deepest needs on a superficial level. And there are many more avenues for distraction on your cell phone. Anyone who needs to get in touch with you can send you a message via text, a messaging app, a social media platform, or email. We are truly wired for connection, so we have the urge to check and respond often. When we see a new message—or when we even see or hear a notification promising one—a dopamine hit is released. This instantly rewards the craving to connect.

And think about what is on the other side of your phone: *literally the entire world*. Any new hobby you want to learn, shopping carts to every store you want to visit, every news channel broadcasting the latest information, every recipe you need for meal planning, every silly video of someone and their dog: it's all there for your enjoyment. (And if you are an Etsy regular like me, you're screwed.) It's fun, it's mindless, and it's far easier than doing whatever mundane or hard thing is in front of you.

It's also far more dangerous than you'd think. When we are occupied by these mindless things, we often do not pay attention to those normal things that could make us feel content—things that we experience *every single day*. The first taste of your morning coffee, the way your partner's eyes crinkle when they smile, the sound of your child's belly laugh, the brushstrokes of color as the sun sets—the list goes on. These lovely little things have great power to influence our moods—but only if we focus on them.

Attention is a limited resource. One of the best studies that demonstrate this is the monkey business illusion by Daniel Simons at Harvard University. If you haven't seen this, don't read on. Stop for a minute and search for "monkey business illusion video" online. (I *said* don't read on.)

Did you watch it? Amazing, right? In the experiment, we see several people passing a ball back and forth. We are asked to count the number of passes the players wearing white shirts make. In the middle of the video, a large gorilla walks out into the center of the circle, thumps its chest, and walks off. Once you know he's coming, it's pretty obvious, but I missed it the first time. Apparently, more than 50 percent of people do. If we are paying attention to one thing, we can clearly miss some very big things! If you knew the gorilla would be showing up, you, like many viewers, likely missed some of the smaller details that change. The experiment demonstrates a concept known in the field of psychology called *inattentional blindness*: the failure to notice what is very visible simply because we aren't paying attention.

Some of those big and very visible things involve people. One summer night my husband and I were sitting out by a campfire chatting with some friends. In the middle of the conversation, one friend pulled out his phone and started reading. (I've learned since then that this is called *phubbing*: snubbing with your phone.) Our friend jumped in and out of the conversation, distractedly, and he seemed not all that invested in what was being said. I know all of you have experienced this at some point. This friend is kind, fun, and not in the least bit rude. I just don't think he realized the impact of what he was doing on everyone else. We pull out our phones so often when we are alone that we may not even realize when we are doing it in public. We also lose track of how long we spend on our phones, and we may be oblivious to the effect that has on others around us. Have you ever turned on your phone to search for just one thing . . . and then completely forgotten what you were trying to find? This jumping on and off our devices has dangerous consequences on our ability to focus and even on our long-term memory.

You may be sick of hearing about neural pathways by now, but what we do and what we think are so directly related to them that I need to talk about them again. If we allow for distraction time and again and if we switch focus constantly, we create a distracted brain that literally will not know how to focus well.

When we shift our focus from one thing to another, we leave a residue of attention behind on the last thing we saw. So our full attention has not transferred to the next thing in front of us. The flow of neural energy through our brain circuitry is disrupted. If you have ever had a conversation with someone who is looking at their phone but looks up to answer you periodically, you have witnessed this disruption. It takes time to make the shifts, and we just don't have enough time to shift our attention completely when we are changing focus constantly.

Chronic distraction leads to chronic stress, which affects both our ability to do a task well and our capacity to remember it. Stress is linked to both the degeneration of the hippocampus (the brain's memory center) and the impaired functioning of the prefrontal cortex, which affects executive function. Executive function is our ability to organize and GSD (get stuff—that's the nice word—done).

I am a person who takes three tries to leave the house. I have to run back each time for something I forgot. I have the same issue at the grocery store, which is why I am there almost every day. My clients, however, often comment on how well I remember tiny details from their sessions. If they tell me they wore a blue dress and ate oatmeal the morning their dog died, I will remember each detail. Why? At first, I couldn't figure it out either, as I have such a hard time remembering anything outside of sessions unless I write it down. It finally occurred to me: when my client is speaking, I am completely absorbed in one thing. For the entire forty-five minutes, my eyes and ears are focused entirely on them.

How we respond to our phones mimics addiction down to the way our brain stimulates the release of neurochemicals. And the creators of these devices knew of their dangers.

According to Business Insider, Bill Gates did not allow his kids to have cell phones until they turned fourteen, and Steve Jobs prohibited his children from using the newly released iPad. If you have kids who use devices, you understand why they did this. Monitoring the use of devices is our greatest parenting battle.

And we don't actually have to be *on* our phones to be distracted *by* them. Several studies have confirmed just having them nearby is enough to create distraction, fractured attention, and a less enjoyable life experience. One study had one group of women bring their phones, on silent mode and out of sight, into a massage. The other group left their phones in lockers outside the room. The group of women who did not have their phones in the room reported greater satisfaction with the massage. Those who had their phones in the room reported being distracted by the low vibration of a message notification and reported a lower satisfaction with the massage overall. Often hearing a notification triggers curiosity and the urge to check the phone. This leaves you feeling a bit unsettled until that craving to know is satisfied. So much for being able to relax during a massage!

A similar study focused on people and their cell phones in restaurants. One group did not have their phones in view, while the others had their phones in plain sight on the table. The group who did not have their phones on the table reported a greater, more enjoyable experience of the evening than those who had their phones visible. (Test yourself on this one the next time you go out to dinner!)

We have become so connected to our phones that they are almost like phantom limbs. I have had patients report they sometimes think they hear a notification or feel a vibration only to check their phones and realize there was none.

According to the studies—and likely your own experience— this type of distraction prevents us from enjoying pleasurable moments in life. It affects our ability to connect, focus and concentrate, and perform a task optimally. Distraction decreases our contentment, affecting our ability to notice things that would help us experience life in a meaningful way.

THE ANXIOUS MIND

As an anxiety specialist, I can tell you this: it is incredibly hard to find contentment when we are feeling anxious. The CDC recently reported that the percentage of adults with an anxiety or depressive disorder in February 2021 had reached 41.5 percent. According to the National Institutes of Health, that number is even higher for teens. These statistics seem to be increasing each year for both populations. We have talked about social media and how it creates anxiety in users. But frequent, incomplete shifts of thought—whether related to devices, everyday distractions, or multitasking, all of which are normal in our hectic lives—have been proven to create more anxiety and depression. When we can't do a task well or have issues focusing or completing tasks, it creates stress. Stress and anxiety are BFFs.

An anxious mind never lives in the present. It tends to live in the future or the past. An anxious mind always circulates what-if questions, considering every possible negative outcome. It's as if we believe that considering all the worst-case scenarios is one way to prepare for them and even prevent them from happening.

Time and again I have seen anxiety prevent people from living a full life without regrets. Don't get me wrong: anxiety can be helpful in the right doses. It helps us consider outcomes and prepare for eventualities, and on some level, anxiety can help keep us safe. Our minds have actually developed to focus on the negative for good reason. Long ago, early humans needed to scan their environment for danger to stay safe and survive, so those who lived in a more or less constant state of alarm had a survival advantage over those who were more relaxed. So what is called the *negativity bias*—the fact that negative comments and experiences stick with us more than the positive ones do and are harder to shake—makes sense evolutionarily. We often dismiss compliments, but if someone criticizes us, we remember that for years.

Anxiety takes this to a whole new level by preventing us from considering possibilities that could be positive. It's a commonly held belief that 85 percent of the bad things we worry about never happen. I'm not certain that we have an exact number, but studies have confirmed most things we worry about are unlikely to occur. Oh sure, *other* bad things do happen, but they are often the things we *don't* worry about. These are the things that catch us off guard, the events that we didn't see coming. But do you know what? We deal with them.

I would love to walk you through what you can do to heal your anxiety, but that is a long process. Healing anxiety involves identifying core beliefs that we have formed about ourselves and the world that elicit anxiety. This would take time and pages beyond what we have left in this book. But I want to give you at the end of this chapter a simple strategy from cognitive behavioral therapy, proven by research, that will help redirect anxious thoughts. These strategies work far better if we can calm ourselves before we try them. Anxiety will always trigger our fight, flight, or freeze response (the activation of our sympathetic nervous system). This response is great if you are in the woods running from a wild boar but not so great in contemporary life. Constant sympathetic stimulation leads to chronic stress and chronic low-grade inflammation, which we know is linked to cardiovascular disease, cancer, type 2 diabetes, and other conditions.

The good news is that we do have a built-in system that we can turn on to counter this stress response. You just have to do something you have been doing from the moment you came into this world: *breathe*.

JUST BREATHE?

Yes, that's right. It can be that simple. I tell clients all the time that breathing is the key to calm. Our breath and our emotions are so closely intertwined. When we are anxious, our breathing becomes rapid and frantic. When we are calm, it is slow and controlled. When we sob out of desperation, our breath becomes uneven and jagged. We often gasp in fear or excitement. Breath and emotion always go together.

Breathing can be a hard sell, though. My clients often come back with "Yeah, I tried that. It doesn't work." My big and tough male executive clients are the hardest to sell on breathing or meditation as a regular relaxation practice. As soon as I say the word *meditation*, I know they immediately conjure up the image of a suburban yoga mom drinking a vegan kale smoothie in her Lululemons. Not for them—until I tell them Navy SEALs do it too.

Every special forces combat unit knows the power of breathing to regulate emotion. It's one of the techniques they use to center themselves in combat. When Ed was a Navy flight surgeon, I learned a lot about the SEALs. It's unreal what the military puts recruits through even before they are accepted into this elite group. If breathing works for them, it will work for anyone.

One of the breathing techniques the SEALs use is box breathing: a four-second inhale, a four-second hold, a four-second exhale, and another four-second hold. Breathing in this way can bring calm in less than five minutes. In fact, relaxation breathing works for me in just one minute. I do six ten-second breath cycles: one slow four-count inhale, and then one slow six-count exhale. Repeat five more times.

One thing to know for now—and this is key—is that your *exhale* has to be longer than your *inhale*. Think of your holds as part of your exhale, lengthening the breath. This is where many of my clients go wrong. When you breathe deeply from your diaphragm (not your chest) and the exhale is longer, you stimulate your vagus nerve, which modulates a vast number of bodily functions but in this case sends a message to your body that it's time to relax. The vagus nerve activates the parasympathetic nervous system (PNS), which then takes over. You may have heard of the PNS in middle school biology class as your "rest and digest" system. Like any new habit, you need to practice. I'm sure the SEALs don't try out box breathing for the first time in the middle of combat and expect it to work. Much like playing an instrument, doing relaxation breathing taps into muscle memory. If you train and condition yourself, when you try it during a stressful moment, it will be very effective in calming the body and centering the mind.

Breathing is the foundation of mindfulness, which will help alleviate both distraction and anxiety. In fact, mindfulness can rewire our brain to live more fully in the present.

A MIND FULL OF CLARITY

Mindfulness means, essentially, to see clearly. When we observe something mindfully, we suspend judgment and see what is really going on. Our observations and feelings are very often clouded with judgment. For example, when we have to wait in a long line, we might think, *This is so annoying* or *This cashier is the worst.* Instead, if we were to practice mindfulness in that moment of waiting in the checkout line, we would take a few deep breaths to calm down our reactive self. Our parasympathetic nervous system would kick in, and then we could begin to observe. Maybe we notice our shoulders tensing up, so we then relax them to release the tension. Maybe we notice the cashier's brow furrowed by stress, so we then feel some compassion toward her. That compassion then releases a few happy neurochemicals, which relax us further. Maybe we are calmer by that point and can say to ourselves, "This is frustrating not only for me but for everyone." Then we don't feel so alone in our suffering and can put it into a better perspective. Do you see how this can work?

Mindfulness helps us notice things we may not have been aware of because our intense emotions had prevented us from doing so. When we make a practice of this, we begin to change our brain structure so that we become less reactive.

This practice calms us down. It also helps with distraction. We can catch when our mind wanders or when the craving to switch to something else hits. We can pause to redirect and act intentionally rather than react distractedly.

Mindfulness also improves our ability to pay attention to things when we are not stressed, strengthening our "appreciation happiness" abilities. Think of mindfulness as our ability to savor our experiences and relationships. *This* is what it means to live fully and to be present in each moment.

IT'S ANCIENT AND IT WORKS

Mindfulness as a practice goes way back, almost 2,500 years. Buddhism's first step toward enlightenment, *sati*, has several meanings, including "memory," which is connected to the words *mindful* and *thoughtful*. Hinduism speaks of *dhyana*, the practice of meditation in which one can still the mind to become aware of what is coming and going internally. In the Judeo-Christian tradition, the psalmist writes, "Be still and know that I am God." As cultures across the world extract principles from mindfulness, it has changed in its essence from these original practices. Yet mindfulness in whatever form still offers a valuable guidepost for people of all faiths and perspectives.

In each tradition, stillness brings awareness of truth, whether it be experiential, existential, or divine. In the late 1970s, Dr. Jon Kabat-Zinn brought these truths to the West and uncovered a few astounding ones of his own. He researched and developed what's known as MBSR, which is the foundation of most of the current psychological research on the subject today. His

eight-week program offered overwhelming evidence of the efficacy of mindfulness in reducing stress and greatly impacting
well-being.

Kabat-Zinn saw that in just eight weeks, participants who
practiced mindfulness meditation became less reactive to stress
and instead were able to respond more calmly in stressful situations. Sarah Lazar and her colleagues conducted further studies
that confirmed that within eight weeks, people who had never
meditated before had four areas of the brain that *increased*
in size:

1. The area that prevents mind wandering (posterior
   cingulate)

2. The area that helps with learning, memory, and emotion regulation (left hippocampus)

3. The area that helps with perspective shifts, empathy,
   and compassion (temporoparietal junction)

4. The area that produces neurotransmitters that regulate mood and sleep (pons)

After eight weeks of mindfulness meditation, one area of the
brain *decreased*: the right hemisphere of the amygdala, the area
of negative emotion such as aggression and fear.

Lazar's studies also discovered that people who meditated
over a longer period of time had more gray matter in their sensory cortex, enhancing their senses and increasing their overall
awareness. This area helps us experience life more fully, taking

in moments with all our senses. They also had more gray matter in their frontal cortex, which increased their memory and decision-making ability.

The study also reported that fifty-year-old meditators had the same amount of gray matter in their frontal cortex as twenty-five-year-olds generally do. Normally that region of the cortex shrinks as we age, contributing to memory loss, but not in this group. In addition, research has confirmed that those who practice mindfulness report less anxiety, depression, chronic pain, and insomnia.

So how long do you have to meditate to reap these benefits? On average, people in the study reported a twenty-seven-minute practice daily. Other studies have reported even eight minutes a day can result in brain changes toward less reactivity. I've found that even one minute of meditation every couple of hours can be effective in reducing stress and alleviating low levels of anxiety.

GETTING STARTED

There are two ways that I recommend people begin with meditation. One is the actual formal practice of meditation. The other is the informal practice, which can happen during everyday tasks.

The formal practice requires you to be still and to focus on your breath. A good way to begin is to set a timer for eight minutes, sit comfortably and still, and breathe deeply, with a longer exhale.

The informal practice requires you to focus on doing one thing at a time and to think about the details of that task and how you feel in that moment. For example, if you are eating, you simply focus on eating as if you are doing it for the first time. This practice is called *beginner's mind*. You notice how food looks, what the fork sounds like as it strikes the plate, how it feels in your mouth, what it tastes like, and how it feels in your throat as you swallow it. If you are washing dishes, you might notice how the soapsuds cover the dishes, the feel of the warm water flowing over your hands, and the sound of the running water. Use your five senses to describe the experience to yourself mentally, as if you were seeing and experiencing these things for the very first time.

Practicing beginner's mind is one way to slow down and pay attention to details that we often miss. This process heightens our awareness and will help us create neural pathways that strengthen this behavior. When we intentionally make time to do this, we condition our brain for it so that this level of awareness begins to happen organically in other moments. We then get better at observing our feelings when we are stressed, which helps us release them rather than get swept up in them. Mindfulness also helps us begin to notice those pleasurable, everyday things that we would miss if we were stressed, hurried, or distracted. Today I found contentment noticing the naughty twinkle in my daughter's eyes; the soft, comforting feel of the blanket at the foot of my bed; the minty taste of peppermint in my afternoon tea; and the song of newly hatched baby birds nestled in my front-door wreath. Life is far from perfect, and stress abounds, but noticing these things brings me moments of peace and even joy.

Meditation takes practice. As you are learning, try to practice self-compassion when it gets frustrating! Your mind will wander, and that's OK. Bring yourself back to counting your breaths and observing how it feels to breathe. Just a few minutes at a time will make a difference. Once you have that down, add on from there.

TURNING THE KEY

- *Eliminate distraction.* Put away all your devices and close all apps that lead to distraction. Set a timer for twenty minutes and focus on one task for that time period. When it is over, take a short break. Celebrate with a little dance, smile, and tell yourself, "I can do this!"

- *Reduce anxiety.* Pick a regular time each day—perhaps before lunch or another time that is more convenient for you. Do one minute of meditation breathing with a slow four-count inhale and a longer six-count exhale. Open your eyes, take one more inhale, and slowly exhale and think to yourself, *This is calm.*

- *Use this CBT technique.* If you find yourself going to a worst-case scenario, ask yourself, *What would the best-case scenario be? What is another outcome somewhere in between the worst and the best? How often in the past has the worst case happened?* Getting our minds off the worst case and open to other possibilities can help reduce anxiety. Remind yourself of these other scenarios every time this particular anxiety sets in.

CHAPTER 12

Priority and Intention

A few years ago, I was sitting in my office alone, after nine sessions back-to-back, just thinking. That day I had spoken to all types of people—from mothers to business owners to angsty adolescents—each for nearly an hour. Nothing out of the ordinary. This is what therapists do.

Yet that evening, an uneasy feeling washed over me as the thought crossed my mind, *When was the last time I had spoken to my own kids for an hour?* With our comings and goings, an extra hour in the day was nearly impossible to come by. I couldn't recall the last time I had sat down with my kids to just listen to them. This realization deeply troubled me.

I decided to make a list of the things and people most important to me. Ed, my kids, my family, and my friends topped that list. Then I added things I love to do: this included singing, exercising, and entertaining. Next I made a second list by looking at where my time went during the week: what I actually was doing and for how long. Work, things I didn't really care about that I had said yes to, social obligations, and time-wasting distractions composed the majority of that second list.

Studying my two lists, I knew there was a problem. Almost none of my time went to those things I loved to do. This was not how I envisioned my life. Cognitive dissonance is that painful feeling we experience when we perceive an internal conflict or inconsistency between our beliefs and our behaviors. And I had it bad. If the most important people in my life were my priority, why were they getting scraps of my time? Why were they getting only scraps of *me*?

If there is any one thing that I want you to remember from this book, it's this: your time is your most valuable possession. Time is a limited commodity, and we can never know how much of it we actually have.

To learn to live more intentionally, I encourage you to make these two lists by considering the following questions. For your first list, ask yourself, *Who and what is most important to me? What do I love to do?*

Now for your second list, ask yourself, *How do I spend my time during the week?*

Look at how your lists line up. It's not always possible to invest the majority of your time in those things most important to you—especially if your job doesn't make it onto your "most important" list. You can, however, look at what time is left over and how you spend it. This exercise can help you recognize what is important to you and then intentionally set aside some time to live in those areas. When we intentionally make room for the people and experiences that are meaningful to us, we create channels for contentment to flow in our everyday lives. Life does not have to be extraordinary to bring peace, purpose, and fulfillment.

I made some big decisions after clearly seeing on paper what my life *really* looked like. With much prayer, I cut down my patient load in half. This was not a particularly good time to cut back on income, as Ed had just left his very secure job to start his own practice. But it made perfect sense given my list and my own intuition.

I wanted more time with the important people on my list. I decided that I was going to start reading with my kids at night like we used to do when they were younger. We picked the book *Wonder* by R. J. Palacio and began to read it together in the evenings. One kid always fell asleep by the end of the chapter each night. Sometimes I did too, and apparently I developed the ability to sleep-read. We loved that time together and started to talk about the themes of the story outside of our reading hour. Several books later, we are still talking.

I also started scheduling a date with my husband every few weeks. Some nights we dressed up and enjoyed a nice dinner out, but more often than not, our date simply consisted of an early morning walk around our neighborhood. Starting my day with someone I love while watching the world awaken around me brings an overwhelming sense of peace and gratitude. There is nothing I want in these moments; I simply savor all that I have. If contentment could be defined in moments, my everyday morning walk would be one of them.

Did my small changes fix my macrolevel problem? Not entirely, but it was a start. Simply allocating a little bit of time in my week to the people who are important to me changed how I felt about my life. What happened in those moments?

Connection, gratitude, mindfulness—and we now know the benefits of all of those. Even with my scattered memory, I can look back on these moments and recall them with unusual clarity. Why? I'm sure you have an idea by now. Our brains are designed to remember experiences that reward us. If we are paying attention and present, we will likely remember these significant times. We can train our minds to gather and store these heart-filling moments. Even amid great challenges, our lives can be tightly held together by countless threads of contentment.

THE NONNEGOTIABLES

I'm not going to tell you how to organize your time or mandate what should be on your "most important" list. I will say that if self-care is not a priority, you are doing yourself and everyone around you a major disservice.

I'm not talking about getting a mani-pedi every week. When I'm talking about self-care with a patient, yes, that list might include things they enjoy. First, however, we have to go through a checklist of essential behaviors—things that make us feel like functioning, normal humans. When these practices are lacking, people feel constantly overwhelmed and stressed. Self-care essentials for optimal mental and physical health include the following.

Sleep. I cannot overemphasize the importance of getting seven to nine hours of sleep a night. In certain seasons of life—like having a new baby or completing a large work project—this is nearly impossible. Hopefully that's just for a season, however, and we can try to get close to those nightly numbers as soon as possible.

Not sleeping is an unhealthy badge of honor in our culture, proving our unwavering fortitude through accomplishment. *I had so much to do, I hardly slept last night.* Our hustle culture often prevents us from prioritizing sleep. Yet it is essential to our ability to live life well. Our brains and bodies were not created to go, go, go. We need a period of time to restore and heal every day.

For most of my life, I have been a five- to seven-hours-a-nighter. After reading numerous studies, I *made the choice* to do less and sleep more. What is the point of accomplishment if we are too tired or unhealthy to enjoy any of it? Constant sleep deprivation is serious and related to a greater risk of heart disease, kidney disease, high blood pressure, diabetes, stroke, and obesity. It absolutely correlates to increased symptoms of anxiety and depression too.

Exercise. Hear me out on this one. Exercise has been proven an effective preventative measure for both anxiety and depression in adults and adolescents. When clients who don't like exercise begin to incorporate it into their daily lives, I've seen energy levels, self-esteem, and outlook on life improve *without fail.* I insist that my clients coming off meds have a regular exercise plan in place. Research tells us that unlike medication, which benefits some and not others, exercise is a mood elevator that will work for everyone.

You have to find the type that works for you, so try different things at first. If you never have exercised, start with a walk—ten to fifteen minutes a day. That's it. Add a few more minutes each week and build to thirty to forty-five minutes three or four times a week. Walking also is a great way to clear the mind, especially first thing in the morning. I have countless clients who never exercised who now can't live without it. The benefits will speak for themselves.

Nutrition. Especially as you get older, you can't expect to put junk in your body and feel great. Nutrition affects mood and health. Period. As you know by now, I love sugar, but I also no longer eat a ton of it because it creates such energy highs and lows. I personally don't want a life completely without sugar, but I have seen that eating healthy foods makes one feel clearer, more focused, and ultimately more content.

Downtime. Scheduling time for rest and relaxation is important. Ask yourself, *What do I need right now?* Sometimes self-care involves connection—going to lunch or taking a walk with a friend. Sometimes it involves relaxation—taking a bath, reading a book, or taking a luxurious nap. Self-care can also include taking a break to do the things you enjoy, like playing golf, baking your favorite cookies, or watching a movie. If you can't think of anything, do an internet search for "100 self-care practices." Scheduling time once a week makes a difference, and even fifteen to twenty minutes a day of something you enjoy can be life changing. Test me on this!

Fun. We often neglect to make time for the things that bring us joy. And yes, I say *make* because that time will never magically appear. Do you love being creative? Playing ultimate Frisbee? Dancing in your bedroom for no reason? Engaging in the activities we enjoy replenishes us, fulfills us, and prevents us from feeling depleted.

Interestingly enough, when I ask my female clients what do they like to do for fun, many of them don't know. My male clients usually have a better idea, but women often sit in silence in my office when I ask this question. There is a larger conversation as to why this is, but most women I speak with say they don't have time for fun. Sure, they might have a glass of wine with their girlfriends and enjoy it, but that's about it.

What could you do that energizes you and makes you feel like you are really living? If you have no idea, start by putting on music that lifts your spirits while you go about your life. It's amazing how great music can elevate any experience and make it more fun.

When we have fun, we feel alive. We see the best version of ourselves and those around us. Fun is a type of self-care. So what prevents us from enjoying life in this way? In my fifteen-plus years of working with women, I've learned that the biggest reason is guilt. If guilt is holding you back, ask yourself, *Where did I inherit the message that I don't deserve to take time for myself? Who told me, either in words or by their actions, that I shouldn't enjoy life?* If you feel guilt, there may be self-worth issues that you need to explore. These habits ensure that your basic human needs to function are met, so life becomes more enjoyable. Hear me: you deserve to live a healthy life that you enjoy.

Put on your own oxygen mask first. How can we take care of children, a spouse, or an aging parent if we ourselves are depressed or empty? I love the saying "You can't pour out anything from an empty cup." If we are filling those around us, we have to be filled ourselves.

If you have children, you have the chance to model healthy living for them. Do you want them to live a life that is all work and no play? Kids are constantly watching and taking notes in the form of creating pathways to cement what they are seeing. Is what they are seeing in you healthy?

What I have listed here are the very basics of prioritizing your mental, emotional, and physical health. Self-care alone won't help you solve deeply rooted issues. If you find you need the type of self-care that constantly compels you to escape the life you are living, you have to see what's underneath—what's causing you to live a life you need to run away from. A few massages ain't going to fix that.

THE YEAR OF NO

Sometimes our own depletion is the result of our inability to say no. I have treated many a yes-man and yes-woman for overwhelming stress and anxiety because they just couldn't say no to people. I wish "people pleasing" were an official diagnosis listed in the *Diagnostic and Statistical Manual of Mental Disorders* because we need to treat it like an illness.

What makes you say yes to things you don't care about? Is it fear of disappointing people? Worry that people will think less of you? If you were in the position of asking the very same thing of someone else, how would you react if they told you no? You'd accept their answer, right? It's amazing how much grace we have for other people and how little we have for ourselves.

Saying yes to the things that aren't that important to us inevitably means saying no to the things that are. Your yeses are as finite as your time. Use both wisely. So if you spend your yeses on things of lesser value, you will sacrifice them elsewhere.

Several years ago, I decided I was going to have a year of no. I wanted to say yes to those people and experiences most valuable to me, and I realized I couldn't do this if I used up all my yeses on things that weren't. This was one of the most freeing moments of my life. If people didn't like me for it? Well, then they weren't my people to begin with. My people—the people I saved my yeses for—loved me for it.

Just because it's good doesn't mean it's a go. Just because you *can* doesn't mean you *should*. We simply are not called to do everything. We need discernment to know what we are called to take on, and then we can prioritize those things. Sometimes we have to let go of good things to make room for great things. Those great things may not be big and flashy, but they are the things that bring meaning and purpose if we consciously make room for them.

And saying yes to everything will at some point foster resentment. If you frequently feel resentful, there is likely a boundary that needed to be set somewhere in your life that was not. That boundary may have been a complete no to some commitment, or it may have been some agreement that did not require so great a sacrifice on your part. There are many ways to set boundaries that take into account your needs as well as the needs of others. For example, say your relatives want to visit on Wednesday. You knew Wednesday was going to be a crazy busy day, but you agreed to have them over for dinner that night. At the end of the day, you felt resentful and exhausted. Perhaps you could have said, "I would love to have you over, but we just can't make Wednesday work with our schedule. Would Friday or Monday be possible?"

I'm a big believer in the idea that we teach people how to treat us. Setting boundaries teaches people that we have limits that they need to respect in order to be in a healthy relationship with us. This limit setting is both self-compassionate and compassionate. It is far easier to be loving and kind when we aren't exhausted or resentful. People who like to control you to get their needs met won't like boundaries. They will push back and fight them. But that's not a healthy relationship, is it? Normal, yes. Healthy, no.

Intentional boundaries help us protect those things and people that are on our top priorities list. They also provide a safeguard around our time and energy. Sometimes we need boundaries with people who drain the life out of us. Sometimes we need boundaries around what is important to us so that we can sustain these life-giving practices. Saying no is one way to set a boundary around our time. Another way to set a boundary around our time is by eliminating distractions.

BREAK UP WITH YOUR DEVICE

Breaking up is hard to do, but that's exactly what I had to do with my phone. Remember that my family was on me for spending more time with my phone than them? When I checked the screen-time report in the settings of my phone, I knew they were right. My phone was the unworthy recipient of more time than I ever imagined. So I decided that the apps that consumed the most time had to go, at least for a while. For me, that meant Instagram and Facebook. I deleted the apps and decided to go on a social media fast for three weeks.

Like any habit, breaking up with devices takes time. We have to train our brains to think differently so we can do differently. These questions help bring a new perspective to this seemingly harmless waste of time:

- What else could I do with the time I would have if I didn't spend it on my phone? (Remember all the things you say you don't have time for, like meditation or self-care? Well, you will have time for them if you take a break from your phone.)

- What makes me want to go on my device? What am I looking to do or see? Am I seeking validation in some form?

- What am I feeling when I sense the urge to go on my phone? It's important to identify the craving that precedes the phone checking so we can recognize it. Have a go-to action planned instead. Take some deep breaths, jump up and down, take a quick walk, drink a glass of water, read something inspiring, pray for someone. In short, do something to replace that mindless check-in.

- What can I tell myself when I want to go on my phone to remember why I'm doing this? A go-to thought or reminder can motivate us to take different actions. I told myself that wasting time here means less time for my family, and that thought helped.

So what happened after three weeks of very limited social media? More than I expected. I stopped caring so much about what other people were doing. I still cared about them, but I wasn't as interested in what they posted for dinner or where they went that weekend. I started to invest in my own *real life*, not the world that I had created on my profiles. I paid more attention to the people around me and listened more intently when they were speaking to me about something. (I know this because the kids called me *Mother* far less. That's what they call me in loud, obnoxious voices when they know I'm not listening.)

I also got more done—a *lot* more, like chapters of this book! I also felt far more peaceful. There is a pervasive, low-level anxiety that accompanies the constant need to check anything. No longer did that nagging feeling have much control over me.

Any time one of my clients is feeling disappointed or frustrated with their life, I recommend a social media fast. No client has ever come back from this exercise saying it didn't help. We only realize how powerful our phones are when we walk away from them.

I try to use my phone more consciously now. I set time limits on certain apps, which you can do on most devices. Once you reach the limit, the app automatically locks up.

It is far too easy to get sucked down a rabbit hole and forget why you even went on your phone in the first place. Try asking yourself these questions: What am I looking for? What do I need to know? Do I need this information right now?

That last question is so important. Often the answer is no. You can wait—especially if you are driving. If it is something important, dictate a note into your phone or write it down as soon as you are safely able so you can go back and address it later. Then fully focus on whatever you are doing in that moment. This takes some intention, but it is well worth it. At the end of the day, we are talking about creating more time in your day for the things and people that ultimately lead to a life of contentment.

TURNING THE KEY

- What is one thing you could do to care for yourself better this week? Maybe it's more sleep, exercise, connecting with a friend, or doing something you love. Write down one thing, and block off time in your schedule to do it. Even one thing this week is a win.

- After you do that one thing, write down in your journal how you felt. If you are not a journal person, stop for a moment to pay attention to how you feel after completing that thing.

- Now pick another thing to schedule for tomorrow or next week. Remember, even fifteen or twenty minutes of doing something you enjoy can increase feelings of calm and contentment.

CHAPTER 13

Resilience

One December evening in 2004, I turned on the local news on the television in my kitchen as I began preparing dinner. The somewhat mindless chatter made me feel less alone as I waited for my husband to return after a long day of residency. At 5:00 on that dark winter night, I stopped what I was doing and watched a story unfold on the screen. I slowly absorbed the details of what had just happened less than an hour away from where we lived in Queens on roads that I knew well.

Victoria Ruvolo was driving home from her niece's vocal recital when three teenagers in a stolen car threw a twenty-pound turkey at her car: a violent, random prank with tragic results. The turkey crashed through her windshield and shattered her face. Ruvolo's passenger managed to grab the steering wheel and guide the car to safety. After she was rushed to the hospital, doctors began the arduous task of putting her face back together. She spent two weeks in a medically induced coma. With every bone in her face crushed and a caved-in esophagus, she was left with a traumatic brain injury. The doctors told her family the brain damage could be permanent and that it was highly unlikely that she would ever resume her independent life.

Months later, I heard that this woman made a full recovery. But I never learned her whole story until I started researching resilience nearly seventeen years later. Victoria Ruvolo was no stranger to adversity. As a teenager, she had suffered the loss of two brothers at different times. Nine years before her own accident, she endured the anguish of losing a long-awaited child through miscarriage. She never had children after that.

Victoria knew pain well, but she also knew how to get through it. Eight months after the near-fatal accident, after extensive reconstructive surgery and months of cognitive and physical rehabilitation, she returned to her job.

I don't believe in a hierarchy of pain and suffering. Pain is pain, relative only to the one enduring it. I have seen, however, some patients move through unbelievably tough situations with life-changing consequences. And I have watched others remain stuck for years in events that, on the surface, don't appear as difficult. So what is it that enables some people to recover from tragic, traumatic situations while others do not?

The answer: resilience.

Psychologists often define *resilience* as the ability to adapt well to hardship, trauma, tragedy, and other challenges. Resilience and how to get it are multifactorial. Resilience is how well someone can "bounce back" from tough life experiences. I don't think that's all though. What I have seen in my practice and life looks more like this: true resilience allows one to move through adversity, absorbing what has happened and emerging with greater insight, strength, and courage.

But there is more to Ruvolo's story. You see, Ruvolo continued to shock not only her doctors but the world. At the trial of Ryan Cushing, the young man who had hurled the turkey at her windshield and was responsible for her senseless suffering, she asked for a more lenient sentence. Cushing could have served twenty-five years in prison for first-degree assault, among other offenses. But thanks to Ruvolo's power of persuasion, he served six months with a five-year probation.

"I didn't want him to rot in jail," she said. "I couldn't see how locking him up for twenty-five years was really going to help him."

Prior to the sentencing, Ruvolo asked questions about Cushing to better understand him. Ruvolo died in 2019, and soon after her death, the *New York Times* reported that she wanted to know: "What could possibly have built up inside him so bad that he had to throw something so hard?"

Seeing a difficult situation from another person's perspective is a hallmark of resilient people. Ruvolo learned that Cushing's father had recently left his mother for another woman. Due to a serious visual impairment, Cushing could not play sports or drive a car. Because Ruvolo could see from another person's perspective, she did not become entangled in her anger or resentment. Instead, she was able to demonstrate pure compassion for this boy, who was suffering in his own way alongside her.

WHAT MAKES US RESILIENT

I used to think that developing resilience required experiencing intense hardship or tragedy, like Ruvolo did. Yet current research says otherwise. Adverse circumstances—whether grief, loss, disappointment, or setback—are a sure thing for any human. During these times, finding contentment is nearly impossible without resilience.

Here are ten scientifically proven practices that can cultivate resilience in anyone, regardless of life experience. Several of them will look very familiar. Still, don't rush past these. Perhaps one or two specifically could help you build your own resilience.

Self-compassion. Just to review, self-compassion frees us to move through waves of intense emotion rather than be ensnared by them. When we confront our own suffering, we do not allow it to control us. By understanding that others suffer too, we consider others' suffering and perspectives, which makes us feel less alone.

Forgiveness. Acceptance and forgiveness go hand in hand. Like acceptance, forgiveness does not mean condoning or approving the offense. It does not free the offender from consequence. It does not even necessitate continuing in a relationship with the offender. Rather, forgiveness means letting go of the anger, hurt, and resentment that can hold the person feeling those negative emotions hostage.

Getting to a forgiveness mindset can take time. Some people may need to heal first, while some find healing through forgiveness. The opposite of forgiveness is ruminating over the event or person, which we know has a negative impact on one's physical and mental health and well-being. Ruvolo credited forgiveness as the path to releasing the intense anger she initially felt.

Facing fears. If you are fearful of an experience, person, or thing, you can build resilience by facing your phobia. Working with a professional to systematically confront fear can be very helpful. Research says exposure therapy, in which you are gradually exposed to the fear incrementally over time, has been proven to build greater courage and strength. Cognitive therapy has also been proven to build resilience by helping someone find fewer negative perspectives to consider. Courage naturally flows out of the ability to conquer that which has controlled us.

Changing your narrative. By exploring our own stories, we begin to develop different perspectives on what happened to us. Good therapy helps do this. We are not often great historians of our own past. Rewriting the narrative gives us insight into the other sides of our experiences.

A few years ago, I decided to do this. When I begin a new project, self-doubt sometimes appears: *You are not smart enough.* I realized that it had to do with my grades in high school; I never felt that I did as well as I could have, and that led me to question my intelligence back then and occasionally now. Therapizing myself, I asked, "What prevented me from focusing more on my academics?" At forty years old, I realized that when I was in boarding school, I spent a lot of my free time talking to other students about their problems and helping them find solutions. I was the girl people came to when they needed help. Although these informal counseling sessions for friends took up valuable time that I could have used for studying, these experiences also equipped me to do what I was ultimately called to do. This exploration finally freed me from a limiting belief that had held me back for decades.

Research confirms that expressive writing provides insight and perspective to help develop flexibility in how we think about ourselves. Participants who wrote their thoughts and feelings about a significant event for four days felt healthier six weeks later and happier three months later.

Flexibility also enables us to find silver linings or positive moments amid struggles. Flexibility overrides all-or-nothing thinking and creates a growth mindset. It enables us to see a situation as both/and. For many, the coronavirus pandemic confirmed this. *Being on lockdown was inconceivably exhausting and isolating* and *I also enjoyed the slower pace and time with my family*: we can acknowledge feeling two seemingly opposing emotions at once.

When we consider our narratives, we must explore the hard emotions; no one needs more toxic positivity, which occurs when we try to bypass these feelings and mask them with affirmations. But once we do work through them, we may be able to consider the good that came from that negative experience. Studies show that people who wrote about three positive things in their day for three weeks reported feeling more engaged with life—in addition to a decline in their pessimistic beliefs—than those who just wrote about their day. If you are a glass-half-empty person—this exercise is for you!

Mindful meditation. Since you've made it this far in this book, you are more than aware that mindfulness helps us take notice and pay attention. That is incredibly helpful when we are looking for the positive. We also know a practice of meditation makes us less reactive, down to changing the neural structures in our brains that foster calmness anytime but especially in the face of adversity. Studies have shown that people who did a mindfulness exercise before looking at disturbing images of a car accident experienced less negative emotion than those who did not do the exercise. Mindful meditation can be that effective that quickly.

Gratitude. Remember the day I got locked out of my house and had to drive an hour away to get a key when I should have been writing? Was I frustrated? Yes, but I *made a choice* to focus on gratitude. Writing is quite isolating, and I was grateful to have had a break that morning to spend with my friend on our walk. I felt grateful that I had a property manager who had an extra key. I was grateful that this happened at the time that it did and not as I was leaving for home. Although my wallet was in the house, I was grateful that I could use my phone to buy a coffee at Starbucks. I was grateful that since I had the extra time in the car, I could listen to one of my favorite preachers give an inspiring sermon that lifted my spirits.

Practicing gratitude that day did not prove as difficult as it would have been had it not already been a regular practice. Gratitude helped me let go of the stress, find the silver lining, and power through the rest of the day. That's everyday resilience.

Building connections. We've already examined how vital connection is to contentment, but knowing we are not facing life alone also builds resilience. Resilience is strengthened when we perform acts of kindness for other people, be it random acts or organized through regular volunteering.

The World Happiness Report from 2020 revealed that one of the reasons we saw an increase in happiness that horrific year was because across the country, people were doing innumerable, generous acts of kindness and caring for strangers. Seeing people do extraordinarily kind and often sacrificial things for one another that year literally strengthened our spirits. These connections gave us all the will to keep going in what was the hardest year imaginable.

Embracing the positive. My friend Kimmy is one of the most resilient people I know—and likely one of the most positive too. Energetic and vivacious, Kimmy has a joy that's contagious and affects everyone around her. A few years ago, Kim lost her mom and her dad several months apart, each unexpectedly. An only child and recently divorced, Kim still stayed positive in the face of unbearable grief.

I called her one day, thinking I would check in and try to offer a little comfort. Amazed by her gratitude for my call, I asked her, "Kim, how do you stay so positive? What brings you peace right now?" I'll never forget her response:

Niro, what brings me peace is imagining my mom meeting Jesus face-to-face and experiencing joy that no earthly human can comprehend. I just imagine her being filled and surrounded with so much light, love, and joy. What brings me peace is remembering playing her the song "You Are My Sunshine" when she was in the hospital. She smiled and sang along when I played it. She sang it to me anytime I was sick or needed comfort. What is also bringing me peace is the idea that she brought me into this world, and I helped usher her out. That I had the gift of forty-one years with her. Everyone at the hospital keeps saying how amazing and strong and dignified I am, and I just say it is all because of her.

This, friends, is what resilience looks like. Psychologists believe we need a 3:1 ratio of positive to negative daily thoughts not only to build resilience but also to *thrive in life*. If we intentionally look for something positive, we will find it, which creates the pathways to develop a more optimistic brain. Optimism directly correlates with resilience, leading to many positive outcomes, including goal achievement.

Self-care. Research shows that we need healthy self-care routines to build resilience. In fact, studies have shown that spending time fosters resilience. Right before I locked myself out of my house that day, I had taken a break from work to walk by the ocean on a cold but sunny afternoon. Being outside and connecting with the beauty of the water absolutely affected my mood, enabling me to get into a more positive mindset more quickly. The research reports twenty minutes outside in nice weather leads to a proresiliency mindset. This type of expansive and open thinking allows us to consider the possibilities, learn from mistakes and failures, seek challenges, and take risks. I think most people—especially us frozen New Englanders—would tell you we feel better in nicer weather. Clearly the benefits are more powerful than we may realize.

Rest. We need not just active rest but *do-nothing* rest. Yes, you overachievers, *nothing*!

Research shows that our brains are quite active when we are *not* doing anything. MRI and PET scans show that the brain "at rest" is significantly active in the areas that affect decision-making, memories, and the processing of emotionally important events.

Scientists explain that during these rest times, the brain is using energy to process our experiences and any new information we have received to create new synaptic pathways. These connections then improve our ability to make decisions and problem solve. They increase our ability to see and think clearly. This is why rest and mental breaks, especially during times of stress, are incredibly vital to our functioning.

RESILIENCE BENEFITS OTHERS

Regardless of what you have gone through—whether you have had a hard life or a relatively easy one—you can cultivate resilience through these practices. This truth is especially important for our kids.

The other day, one of my friends exclaimed how ridiculous it was that our local high school offers a class on "adulting." I disagreed and explained that a class like that is necessary because adolescents are not developing the resilience to manage adult tasks and stressors. When they get to college and run into a challenge, they want to quit and come back home or transfer schools. This lack of resilience is, in part, also why we are seeing rates of anxiety and depression skyrocket in younger populations. "OK, but how did we even get here?" she said, shaking her head in disbelief.

If you are a parent reading this book, yes, it is our fault. If we want our kids to build resilience, we have to teach them how. First, we have to model resilience for them. Kids have a very sensitive BS meter for the discrepancies between our actions and words. We can't just say we have to do something. We need to teach them how to "do" resilience, meaning we can't do everything for them. They have to fail if we want them to learn how to recover from failure. They have to feel disappointment if we want them to learn how to pick themselves up from it. Stepping back and teaching kids the practices that build resilience offer scientifically based solutions to this pervasive problem.

Resilience not only benefits you; it has the power to strengthen and heal those around you. What would the world look like if we dared to step into the power of these practices?

Cushing learned that Ruvolo, the victim of his careless prank, had insisted that he receive a much shorter sentence than the system of law would have meted out. As he stopped in the courtroom to speak to Victoria, he began weeping uncontrollably. Victoria embraced him, gently touched his face, and patted his back as one would a wayward, beloved son.

"I'm so sorry," he said to her as he sobbed. "I didn't mean it."

"It's OK, it's OK," Victoria replied. "I just want you to make your life the best it can be."

And he did. Two months later, Cushing told her that it was her ability to forgive that changed his life. Now Cushing is a working, productive member of society. He speaks to kids about the mistakes that he made.

He has become Victoria Ruvolo's legacy.

TURNING THE KEY

- Reread the ten practices of resilience in this chapter. Ask yourself, *Which of these areas that build resilience is challenging for me?*

- Pick one area and commit to one practice a week for the purpose of building resilience. Perhaps it is looking for three positive moments each day, or performing an act of kindness, or taking a walk outside. Perhaps it is considering what it would take to forgive or resting and doing nothing for twenty minutes. Feel free to think of your own. Choose one. Start small.

- Think of the best time in your day to do this. Write it down in your schedule or on a sticky note to post where you can see it.

- After you do it, tell yourself, "This is strengthening my mind and spirit," or think of another motivating statement that resonates with you.

CHAPTER 14

Faith

This last key might be a bit controversial. Plenty of people who do not have strong ties to any faith tradition feel contented. Numerous studies over the years, however, strongly suggest that religious people are indeed happier and healthier than the nonreligious.

Interestingly enough, when we look closer at the results of these particular studies, we see that a connection to God does not seem central to happiness. Is it faith and a connection to the Divine that leads to contentment? Or the things that often come along with religion—community, a sense of purpose, and calming rituals?

I want to differentiate between religion and faith because you can certainly have one without the other. Religion is organized. It usually involves a people group that shares a belief system, practices, traditions, and rituals. Faith, on some level, is inexplicable. I think of faith as a trust and confidence in a supreme being, a trust that is sustained by an ongoing and dynamic relationship. The ancient Greek manuscript that Christians know as the Epistle to the Hebrews defines faith as the "confidence in what we hope for and the assurance about what we do not see." Unlike science, which is founded on objectivity, faith is not. We cannot see it or measure it. Although you can find commonalities in the faith experience, the beauty of faith is that, like any good relationship, it is personal and unique to that individual and God. For that reason, it can be quite distinct from organized religion.

In best-case scenarios, religion fosters a stronger and more tangible faith experience. But of course, this is not always the case. Many people have suffered religious trauma, which has turned them away from faith altogether. Even the idea of God can become a trigger. I'm here to tell you that religion and faith are not one and the same. When I refer to faith in the conversation on contentment, I mean an individual connection with an all-knowing, compassionate, and ever-present God.

ARE RELIGIOUS PEOPLE REALLY HAPPIER?

Like I said, the answer to that question is hard to decipher. One study examined data from the World Value Study, which surveyed people in one hundred countries over a span of forty-three years. The results concluded that Protestants, Buddhists, and Roman Catholics were more satisfied with their lives than Jews, Hindus, and Muslims. Nonreligious people fell somewhere in between them and Orthodox Christians, who were found, according to this study, to have the lowest rates of happiness.

Skeptical? I sure was. That just didn't make sense to me, because I have known people from every one of those religious groups, here and abroad, who are happy—as well as people from every one of those religious groups who are *unhappy*. Yet the study was quite comprehensive and took place over a long period of time.

It's hard to isolate religion without taking into consideration other social factors that affect well-being. This study also revealed that a person's financial stability, health, freedom of choice, and control over life also had to do with the rankings and were tied into certain populations surveyed.

More recent studies report that socioeconomics and politics played a major factor in the correlation between religion and happiness. In other words, the more money and freedom people had, the less religion had an impact on their happiness. Residents of countries that are less developed and who face more life challenges and stressors appeared to rely on religion for hope and comfort. The outlier, however, proved to be the United States. Even though the United States is considered to be economically stable and democratic, religion appears to make people happier here.

What numerous studies confirm is that the benefits of religion center on the fact that it usually provides community. If you have made it to this chapter, you know the value of connection and its impact on well-being. A community of people with shared values and perspectives creates an even stronger bond between its members than groups that do not share similar beliefs.

Interestingly enough, most religions also encourage collective group singing or chanting. And did you know it is nearly impossible to be anxious and sing at the same time? Due to the numerous physiological processes singing involves, our brains can't handle doing both simultaneously. A woman who attended one of my talks in which I mentioned singing as a strategy to combat anxiety sent me an email a few days later saying, "It actually works!" Three days after this event, her car spun out in a terrible blizzard. Terrified, she mustered up the courage to get back on the road behind a snowplow. She credits singing loudly all the way home as the reason she stayed calm.

Singing releases both endorphins and oxytocin and has been proven to reduce anxiety. Group singing is one of the most powerful human emotional experiences because we feel the mood-elevating benefits of singing *and* connection. Group singers experience a range of positive emotions, from calm to exhilaration. One study even found that singers have lower levels of cortisol, leading to better health and lower stress. Where can you find hundreds of not-so-gifted singers joyfully belting out songs together every week? Church.

Through religious communities of all kinds, members find connection as an expression of altruism, compassion, gratitude, support, and belief in a higher power that fosters the acceptance of hardships. Clearly religion encompasses many of the practices that we know scientifically boost mood and ensure well-being.

But what about God? Does a connection to a divine Spirit lead to contentment? Does God make a difference?

YOUR BRAIN ON GOD

Neuroscientists have often wondered if we are hardwired for faith. Is there some indication from what we know about the intricate workings of the brain that God indeed exists? Neurotheology is a developing field that uses science to study spiritual practices through brain imagery. Studies in neurotheology show areas of the brain lighting up in response to prayer and other spiritual experiences that trigger our reward pathways and release those happy neurochemicals. Other studies attribute this activation to the psychological comfort that the idea of God provides. Although scientists cannot prove the existence of God simply through brain scans, the discoveries they have made are quite curious and have left them asking more questions. There is little doubt that the brain is designed in such a way to facilitate and promote spiritual practices. And it's not one part of the brain; spiritual experiences involve the whole brain.

One study looked at the parietal lobe, which processes sensory information and helps establish one's sense of self in relation to the world. Scientists found that when someone is engaged in religious experiences, prayer, or meditation, this part of the brain becomes deactivated and essentially shuts down. The boundaries between self and a larger force—God, the universe, or whatever you feel connected to—dissipate and become blurred. That person then begins to feel at one with that larger force.

The frontal lobe helps with focus and concentration and is the executive function center that aids us in making choices. This part of the brain also shuts down during religious or faith experiences, which make us feel as if something is happening to us beyond our own control. If you talk to people of faith, many will attest to the truth of having experiences where things have happened that they themselves did not plan or coordinate. Some of these experiences include a calming peace, an awakening, an increase in knowledge, or a lightness of spirit. You can see from these studies that spirituality has the power to literally quiet the mind.

If you believe in God, it may make perfect sense to you why our brains were created to allow for these experiences. For those who don't, these findings in neurotheology may leave you with many more questions yet to be answered.

Regardless of how many scientific studies or historical documents we have attesting to the veracity of God, I do know this: finding faith requires a step of faith.

Science may be good for answering many questions, but there are some questions that absolutely require faith. We actually take steps of faith every day. Getting married is one of them. There is no scientific experiment that will tell us that this person who we have chosen for life is the "right" one. Hopefully we use both our brains *and* our hearts to make that decision, but there are no guarantees that this will be forever. That step is one of faith. Getting on an airplane is another step of faith. We trust in a pilot we don't know and in a plane we have no control over simply because the odds are in our favor. But again, there is no science in that moment that will ensure that plane you are on will land safely.

In both these situations, we make decisions based on what we know to be true from our experience. We have spent time with the person we are going to marry, and they have shown on some level that they can be trusted. We get on a plane because we have seen that planes are safe. We know certain protocols are taken to ensure safety, including vigorous training for pilots. It is easier to have faith when a person demonstrates over and over that they are worthy of trust. And it is easier to try something when you have done it again and again and felt safe.

A life of faith works much the same way. Initially, faith may seem vague and obscure. How can you develop a relationship with someone you can't see, touch, or hear? When you step into a life of faith, you take a chance, much like you do with any relationship. And like any relationship, only by spending time, listening, and observing will you *really* know if God is trustworthy.

LISTENING TO WISDOM

"Listen to the voice within," "Follow your heart," "Trust your feelings": although I love the sound of these statements, as an anxiety therapist, I find that they create great conflict in me. Feelings come and go and fluctuate. Making a decision in the midst of a wave of emotion can be risky. And I think most of us have experienced following a feeling only to find that at some point, that feeling changes.

When my clients are in the midst of strong emotions, I encourage them *not* to make any big decisions. DBT highlights a principle called the *wise mind*. The research in this modality of therapy states that the mind can be thought of in two parts: the rational mind and the emotional mind. The rational mind, or the brain, is made up of what we know intellectually to be true: our beliefs, the facts, and our reasons based on our experiences. The emotional mind, or the heart, is a deep well of emotion. This part makes decisions based on what "feels right," overemphasizes the validity of emotions, and can get swept away by them. What DBT encourages is to find the meeting place between the two minds—the wise mind—that takes into account the dimensions of both knowledge and emotion. To me this quiet, often hidden place is the home of wisdom.

That meeting place in the middle—the intersection of the mind and heart—is where I believe the voice of wisdom lives. Wisdom speaks firmly, but she is not loud. As we have seen through studies in neurotheology, the brain can quiet itself, which in turn allows us to hear. We all have this capacity biolog-ically, yet so many of us don't make space to listen to this voice. And from working with hundreds of clients and spending time in my own silent listening, I know why.

Silence is hard because the voice of wisdom is honest. She speaks the truth: sometimes words full of peace and joy and sometimes words that we might not want to hear. It's only when we sit in silence that those things, which have sunk to the bottom of the well of emotion, rise to the surface. We can easily ignore the voice of wisdom because she speaks softly. Once she does, though, we cannot unhear. We can run, avoid, and distract, but we cannot unknow. Those words leave an indelible imprint on the soul. No matter how hard the words are to accept, they are always wrapped in compassion and meant to lead us into a life of contentment.

I believe we can all find that sacred space and in it discover the wisdom of the divine Spirit. In this space, I have learned to discern the voice of this Holy Spirit. It is a voice that sounds like my own but I know is filled with divine wisdom, because I have often had thoughts that are vastly distinct from my own thoughts and feelings and yet they undeniably resonate as truth. In that space, there are answers that have been carefully placed to questions we have yet to ask. The wisdom we seek lies patiently, waiting to be discovered. We simply need to ask the questions and listen.

There is nothing I enjoy more than helping people learn to listen and experience this voice, who I call God.

THE GOD OF SMALL THINGS

This is probably a good time to tell you that I hear from God. A lot—like, every day. It's the reason I'm even writing this book. Trust me when I say that when I first learned to discern God's voice in this way, I did not take it lightly. We psychotherapists are highly trained to help people *not* hear voices. But stay with me on this one.

I've been talking with God for a long time. When you have a friend you have known forever, you might know what they might do or say before they do or say it. I recently received a thoughtful gift from a friend, and even before I opened the card, I knew who it was from. When I read the card, I said, "Of course. This is totally Lauren." The gift reflected many facets of her personality *and* what she knew about me. I have said the same of God over and over again, seeing God's handprints and footprints on my life.

Because God has proved trustworthy in my life and because God has comforted me in some of my lowest moments and provided ways that have led to some of my highest, I find meaning and purpose through this relationship like no other.

Spiritual transcendence is one's experience of the sacred that affects self-perception, feelings, goals, and the ability to transcend difficulties. This type of faith offers a lens of understanding through which we see ourselves and the world around us. A large part of faith and a relationship with the divine Spirit is the spiritual transcendence that occurs that helps us find peace, purpose, and contentment.

I have witnessed real miracles from a young age and now into adulthood. I grew up in a family that was open to the miraculous, and I think that made all the difference. Let me also remind you that my parents are physicians, so faith never came at the expense of science. We believe wholeheartedly that they go together. Maybe someday I can tell you those stories. And not everyone has such dramatic stories of how God orchestrated the events of their life. When one is walking the faith journey, God will show up every day in small ways, if we are looking.

People frequently say to me, "The universe is telling me something" or "The universe spoke to me." I believe that God designed this universe, so sure, God can use anything in it to speak to us: a road sign, a random encounter with a stranger, an Instagram post, a friend's text at just the right time, or animals. If we are paying attention, we can see God everywhere. If we aren't, we can miss it—just like we can miss anything significant when we aren't looking. Hearing the voice of wisdom in real time often happens in moments like this.

Once you have seen that the voice of wisdom can be trusted and that God has your best interests in mind, it is easier to take risks and bigger steps of faith when you are led to do so.

I don't believe God to be some sort of genie granting every wish we command. I have prayed many passionate and persistent prayers not answered in the ways I have wanted. I have lost dear friends, seen people I love suffer, and been disappointed time and again by life. Although God didn't give me what I wanted in these situations, God always gave me himself. I can't explain the peace you can feel in these moments, but it truly is a peace that "transcends all understanding" (Philippians 4:7 NIV), one that has left me not with everything I wanted but certainly with what I needed.

WHEN GOD IS ENOUGH

People of faith can often fall into the same traps in their spiritual life as we try to find contentment. I have noticed lately that many Christians hold on to the idea of God doing "immeasurably *more* than all we ask or imagine" (Ephesians 3:20 NIV; emphasis mine). Once again, we hold on to the promise of getting more, which can make it hard to find contentment right in this moment. Can God do more? Of course. Will God work according to what is best for you? Most definitely. Should we pray for our dreams and goals? Without a doubt. Yet many of us are fixated on those goals and dreams and prayers being answered, thinking when that happens, *then* we will be happy. What we often miss is that God enables us to be content right now, in this moment, because the presence of God alone is enough.

This realization—that God is enough—was the reason I stopped taking new patients and cut down my practice in half at a time when, from a financial perspective, I should have kept working to capacity. My decision did not make sense to me, yet it was clearly spoken by the voice of wisdom within me. People repeatedly asked me, "Why are you doing this? What is your end game?" Honestly, I had no idea. But I was getting messages everywhere that I needed to make this change. I also knew I needed more time for my family and for my own mental health.

I had mentioned earlier that God had also revealed to me through that voice that new things lay ahead. I knew I didn't have room to receive them, given how full my life was at that time. It was the voice that led me to craft a book proposal in 2018. Book proposals are grueling, especially when you don't consider yourself to be a writer, yet I knew it was something I had to do. My hope was to get a book deal, but I knew that was really hard too. Having spoken to my friend's literary agent, who advised me to put that written proposal on hold, I started to focus on starting a podcast. Writing was one thing, but talking? A therapist knows how to do that. The podcast, *All Things Life*, features many conversations that helped bring mental, physical, and spiritual healing to a larger audience all over the world.

I remember one day in September hearing that voice say, "It's time." I knew by the excitement in my spirit that God was talking about the book. God gave me a new vision and renewed energy for the book. We were in the midst of the pandemic, and people seemed more discontented than ever before. I knew this message needed to get out, and I decided that even if I needed to self-publish, I would do it. Yet I figured it would be in the future. With four kids learning at home, there was just no time to take on another thing.

Still, about a month later, as I dusted off my book proposal to see if the content was still relevant, I received an email out of the blue. An editor had come across my work and was wondering if I was developing any book proposals. The rest—well, you are looking right at it.

I wish I could tell you that since I cut back on my practice, life has become peaceful, calm, and smooth. I can't. This past year has been the hardest one of my life, taking on the new things that God spoke to me about in addition to the responsibilities of a clinician during a national mental health crisis and being a wife and a mom. I *can* tell you that God has met me every step of the way. Every day has certainly not been happy, but because of the strength God has given me, I have been able to find contentment and peace even in the midst of struggle. In my life, I have found that Jesus has always been enough.

If you find faith—if you make space to hear the voice of wisdom—the rest of the seven keys will naturally flow from this one. It is the way God intended we live this precious life. When you invite God on your journey, God not only enables you to experience contentment but equips you to find deep meaning by leading you in a life of purpose. This purpose may not look worthy in terms of what our culture values. But consider this: What if our true purpose is to just be? What if our divine purpose is to be the tangible embodiments of light, hope, strength, love, and peace? Good things come from a life lived in this way. Those are the real gifts—for us to both keep and give away to each person we meet along the journey.

I would bet my entire career on this: if you are true to *this* purpose, you will find contentment and, regardless of the circumstances, peace. In our world, with all its demands and pressures, peace is priceless.

TURNING THE KEY

- Make a list: write down the questions most pressing to you in this moment, the ones to which you have yet to find answers.

- Take some time to sit and ask the questions one by one in your mind.

- Invite the voice of wisdom—the divine Spirit, who I call God—to speak to you. Listen to see what comes to the surface.

- Know you may receive answers in that time or you may begin to see them as your life unfolds them.

- Continue to sit for a time in silence each day and ask the questions. Write down any information afterward that may have come to the surface.

- This is a process; stay with it and stay open. I know you will find exactly what you need.

Epilogue

There are just a few more things I want to say before we go our separate ways.

I wrote this book as if I were talking to one person: that's you. I care about you. I see you too often caught up in the things that make life harder, less fulfilling. I know those things feel important, even urgent. They consume your time and your energy, leaving less of it for you, for the people you love, and for experiences that really matter.

I love the book *The Alchemist* by Paulo Coelho. (Spoiler alert: I'm about to tell you what happens in this book.) The story takes you on the complex and magical journey of a shepherd boy, Santiago, in search of a hidden treasure he saw in a dream. Along the way, he meets many people that help guide him and move him forward toward his destination. As he gets close to the pyramids, the place where he believes his treasure is buried, he is told to listen to his heart for guidance. His heart speaks of many different things, which is somewhat confusing to him. Yet after an exhausting journey across an entire hot, sun-baked desert, he gets to that spot and begins to dig for this treasure.

As night falls, several men approach him and beat him violently, hoping to take whatever gold they assume he has. Eventually they realize he has nothing, and Santiago tells them he was actually digging for treasure. One of the men laughs and mocks Santiago. He criticizes him for being so stupid as to follow a dream. He discloses that he himself once had a dream while lying in the very place that they were standing near the pyramids. He described to Santiago the place where *his* treasure was buried. But unlike Santiago, he had never pursued it.

That place—the place the man described to Santiago—was on the other side of the desert, at a church, exactly where Santiago started his journey. Santiago knew this had to be a sign. The men disappeared, and, Coelho writes, "the boy stood up shakily, and looked once more at the Pyramids. They seemed to laugh at him, and he laughed back, his heart bursting with joy. Because now he knew where his treasure was." Santiago once again crossed the desert and made the long trip home, back to the church right where he began. There, indeed, he found his treasure.

And so I ask you, Do you know where your treasure lies?

To find it, consider these two questions: *How much does your happiness cost? And is it worth the price you are paying?*

We often sacrifice that which is most valuable to us to attain what we *think* we need to make us happy. When you take a moment to think about what you *really* value, it becomes very clear what matters and what doesn't. Those urgent, pressing desires almost never make that list. Fame, money, power, and material comforts come at a high price. What are you sacrificing to pay for it?

I wrote this book to remind you that you actually have everything you need to find contentment right in this very moment. Much like Santiago, it's been with you in the place where you started all along. If you can't find contentment here, it is very likely that you never will, no matter how much you have. The keys in this book will guide you to find a life full of it.

Finding contentment means making choices. It may mean doing less, spending less, and striving less for what we think will make us happy or what the world tells us we need to feel worthy. Instead, contentment is settling into the things we know bring us peace and a sense of calm. Finding contentment means spending your time meaningfully and intentionally, doing the things you love, and loving those around you fully and completely. At some point, contentment declares that *enough* truly *is enough*.

If we choose to live life in this way, we will not need to find contentment. Contentment will naturally and gracefully find *us*.

You are now equipped with tools that will assist you on your journey and the knowledge and faith to believe that you can do this. You are not alone. Though you may not see them, there are many who are walking this path with you. Remember, too, that you walk this path not only for yourself but for those who surround you, including your children and the generations that come after you. Many people are on this path searching for contentment. You now know how to find it.

Finally, my hope is that you would know that each day is an opportunity for a new start. You may feel like you are starting over, but you aren't. Although Santiago in *The Alchemist* ended up exactly where he started, he was not the same. It was the magic of the journey that made him who he was: a man with great wisdom, strength, and perspective shaped through experience that enabled him to appreciate his real treasure once it was found.

Know if you walk the path one step at a time, one breath at a time, taking in the view as you go, you will most certainly find contentment. You might even find the best version of yourself, above what you could have asked for or imagined.

You now know where your treasure lies.

With much love,
Niro

Acknowledgments

It takes a village to write a book, at least for me. This is my village:

Ed: Forever grateful it was you that night. God knew no one else could be married to me. Saying thank you will never be enough for all you do for me. This book would never have happened without you. I love you with all my heart.

Natalia: The smart girl with the kind heart, who happens to be beautiful too. Keep being exactly you. We need more of what you've got in this world.

Samuel: Your hugs bring healing and make every day a good one. You will always be my favorite son. I hope your wife doesn't mind me coming with you on your honeymoon.

Sofia: My prophet. Share your wisdom with everyone you meet, my fierce, strong girl. Some days it was only your words that kept me going. You are a gift.

Carolina: Everything I knew about parenting clearly didn't matter when you were born. You are proof that life is full of good surprises. Keep being the fire in this family, my sweet girl.

Mom and Dad: I hit the jackpot with you two. Thank you for your energetic, unconditional love and support of everything we do—especially sex talks. You are the definition of compassion.

Krissy and Eddie: You kept me laughing when I needed it most. Krissy, thanks for being the mom they always wanted and needed especially while I was writing. So grateful for you both.

Dushy: Your prayers meant the world to me, and God always speaks through you. You're next!

Sonia T.: Pastor and senior prophet, forever wise. Grateful to travel on this journey with you.

ACKNOWLEDGMENTS

Lucilene C.: You are our family's angel and the sister-friend I needed. I now love broccoli because of you.

Amy Julia B.: Thank you is not enough. You are the real deal, and I'm grateful for thirty-two years of you.

I get by with a little help from these guys:

BATB: You make my life fun. Michaele G.: For your pure heart and loving me for a lifetime—forever grateful for you and the OG. Meg D.: For being the sister I always wanted. Lauren M.: For being my ride or die and always sharing your nachos and tequila. Lisa B.: For being the best wife a girl could ask for. Minnie M.: Your patience and kindness are otherworldly. Debbie C.: For making me laugh even when you don't mean to. Purvi S.: For being that friend who will always watch through the window with me.

Melissa A.: For sharing your precious time, encouragement, and incredible energy. I loved you from the start!

Aimee D.: Soul sister. Here we go!

Danielle C.: For your cards and gifts and for always bringing light even amid your own darkness.

Sandy P.: Seriously the most talented angel and sent from heaven just at the right time. Forever grateful.

Rob S.: For seeing somebody when I felt like nobody. Thank you for always believing.

Dan L.: Likely smartest person I know and the friend I always wanted—thank you.

Marybeth M.: For sharing your wisdom and knowledge.

All my mom friends who dropped off, picked up, fed, and kept my kids on playdates so I could work and for all your encouraging words about this book. I'm so grateful for all of you and your friendship!

To all those who soaked every page of this book in prayer and intention:

All my cousins, especially Shyamo, Sushi, Shala, and John: For your texts, scriptures, and words. I love you all so much.

Bea E.: My anchor. Thank you for staying true to the vision and bringing me back to it when I was drifting.

Craig and Karly H.: Your support, direction, and friendship through every step of this journey have been gold to me.

Carine M.: For your incredible light and shining bright wherever you go.

Jen L.: For thinking of me always and sharing your positivity even when you had every reason not to. You are strength.

Camille M.: For your big heart and for years of cheering me on.

Anna L.: For feeding my body and soul.

Carrie A.: You are a warrior and I love you . . . but don't bring dem goats around here.

A. J. and Mirjam P.: For constantly checking in on me and reminding me I could do this.

My Walnut Hill church family: Anna Mae A., Naa and Bob K., Adam and Carrie D., Brian Mowrey, the Ridgefield Community Group, and the Diversity Team. This is because of all of you.

Jake and Amber: For dealing with my last-minute-ness and still praying for me!

Tarique P.: For sixteen years of making room for my people and being a great teacher.

Chris P.: For generously sharing your time and helping shape the vision.

Valerie W. Z.: For taking a chance on me and truly seeing me. Your compassion and curiosity are unmatched. Grateful for your voice in this book.

To Rachel Reyes, Emily Benz, Jana Nelson, and everyone at Broadleaf Books: A huge thank-you for everything you did to get it right. I'm so grateful for a team with such big hearts to go along with your big talent. I hope I make you proud.

Finally and with much gratitude:

To all my patients over the last sixteen years: Thank you for sharing your life with me. You are my greatest teachers, and I want you to know your healing has healed me too.

Notes

See the references section for full information about sources.

CHAPTER 1: NORMAL

For mass shooting statistics, see Brewster (2021). For the definition of *contented*, see *Merriam-Webster Dictionary* (n.d.).

CHAPTER 2: CRAZY

For material on heuristics, see Henderson (2017). Information on burnout comes from Kelly (n.d.) and NBC News (2020). The World Happiness Report data come from World Happiness Report (2019) and Radu (2019). Happiness and life satisfaction data come from the Pew Research Center (n.d.); Ortiz-Ospina and Roser (2013); and Ortiz-Ospina (2019). Information about suicidal ideation in college kids comes from St. Amour (2020).

CHAPTER 3: CRAVINGS

The information on pleasure comes from Moccia et al. (2018); Taylor (2015); Love (2018); Lieberman and Long (2019); Biggers (2018); Chaudhry and Gossman (2020); and *Psychology Today* (2018). For material on FOMO, see Brustein (2015); *Merriam-Webster* (n.d.); Haynes (2018); Brown (2011); and Buswell (2004). For information about countries and relative happiness, see Matthews (2017); Martela et al. (2020); Moulds (2019); Radu (2019); and Buddhist Centre (2019).

CHAPTER 4: SELFIES

For this chapter, I consulted the following sources: Roman (2014); Diefenbach and Christoforakos (2017); Casale, Fioravanti, and Rugai (2016); Misiner (2017); Mills et al. (2018); Woronko (2015); Pounders, Kowalczyk, and Stowers (2016); Sperling (2020); Griffiths (2018); Luthar and Sexton (2004); Sternlicht and Sternlicht (n.d.); Konrath, O'Brien, and Hsing (2010); Konrath (n.d.); Seppälä (n.d.); Tolentino (2019); American Society of Plastic Surgeons (2019); Parker (2019); SingleCare Team (2021); and Musick (2021).

CHAPTER 5: PARADISE

This chapter's source material includes StuffMirror (2015); Phillip (2015); Oppong (2019); May (n.d.); and McDaniel and Radesky (2017). The Mary Oliver line is from her poem, "The Summer Day" (n.d.).

CHAPTER 6: HABITS

For this chapter, I consulted these sources: Palmer (2021); Stieg (2019); Weinschenk (2019); Duhigg (2014); Icahn School of Medicine at Mount Sinai (n.d.); Clear (2018); van der Weiden et al. (2020); Habits Buzz (2017, 2019); Pressfield (2003); Ford et al. (2018); McKay and McKay (2013); and Ford et al. (2018).

CHAPTER 7: ACCEPTANCE

The sources for this chapter include Chowdhury (2019); Carson and Langer (2006); Herbert and Brandsma (n.d.); and Ford et al. (2018). For the information on gray matter, I consulted Pillay (2016). For the James Baldwin victim quote, see https://www.goodreads.com/quotes/75199-the-victim-who-is-able-to-articulate-the-situation-of.

CHAPTER 8: SELF-COMPASSION

This chapter's sources include Singer and Bolz (n.d.); Braehler and Neff (n.d.); and Neff and Germer (2017). Studies that show links between self-compassion and well-being include Hollis-Walker and Colosimo (2011); Neff, Hsieh, and Dejitterat (2005); Neff, Pisitsungkagarn, and Hsieh (2008); Neff, Kirkpatrick, and Rude (2007); Daye, Webb, and Jafari (2014); Finlay-Jones, Rees, and Kane (2015); Raes (2010); Breines et al. (2014); MacBeth and Gumley (2012); Blatt (1995); and Neff (2003, 2015).

CHAPTER 9: GRATITUDE

This chapter draws from the following sources: Burton (n.d.); World Happiness Report (2019); Greater Good Science Center (n.d.); Brown and Wong (2017); Wood, Linley, and Linley (2020); Brown (2018); and Doyle (2020). For the Alice Morse quotation, see https://www.goodreads.com/quotes/9207779-everyday-may-not-be-good-but-there-s-something-good-in.

CHAPTER 10: CONNECTION

For this chapter, I consulted these sources: Mineo (2017); CDC (2020); Hammond (2018); Monroe (2019); Waldinger (2015); CMHA National (2019); Seppälä (2012); and House, Landis, and Umberson (1988). For information on the need to belong, see Baumeister and Leary (1995); McPherson, Smith-Lovin, and Brashears (2006); Kross et al. (2011); Martino, Pegg, and Frates (2015); Santi (2017); Lohmann (2015); Baltazzi (2019); O'Bryon (n.d.); Baraz and Alexander (2010); Moll et al. (2006); Suttie (2013); Diener and Seligman (2002); Vaillant (2013); Parker-Pope (2009); Shankar et al. (2011); O'Conner (n.d.); Sukel (2019); Kennelly (2012); Poulin (2014); White (2010); Kukk (2017); and Poulin et al. (2013).

CHAPTER 11: PRESENT FOCUS

I relied on the following sources for this chapter: Carson and Langer (2006); Herbert and Brandsma (n.d.); Suttie (2019); Leaf (2020); Vahratian (2021); National Institute of Mental Health (2017); Santos (2020); Weller (2018); Robinson (2020); Lazar et al. (2005); Schulte (2015); Hölzel et al. (2011); Dixon (2017); Powell (2018); Pawlowski (2017); Nazish (2019); Desbordes et al. (2012); Leonard (2020); and Simons (2010).

CHAPTER 12: PRIORITY AND INTENTION

This chapter relies on the following sources: Sharma, Madaan, and Petty (2006); Harvard Health (2019); American Psychological Association (n.d.); and Cleveland Clinic (2020).

CHAPTER 13: RESILIENCE

This chapter's sources include Patel (2014); Arch and Craske (2006); American Psychological Association (2012); and K. Newman (2016).

CHAPTER 14: FAITH

For this chapter, I consulted Newbergh (2019); Septien (2019); Perry (1998); Villani et al. (2019); Neuroscience News (2019); Collins (2018); Ngamaba (2018); Walsh (2017); Marshall (2019); Quinn (2014); Suttie (2020); Keating (n.d.); and Horn (2012).

EPILOGUE

For the epilogue, I referenced Coelho (1993).

References

American Psychological Association. 2012. "Building Your Resilience." https://www.apa.org/topics/resilience.

———. n.d. "More Sleep Would Make Most Americans Happier, Healthier and Safer." https://www.apa.org/action/resources/research-in-action/sleep-deprivation.

American Society of Plastic Surgeons. 2019. "Americans Spent More Than $16.5 Billion on Cosmetic Plastic Surgery in 2018." April 10, 2019. https://www.plasticsurgery.org/news/press-releases/americans-spent-more-than-16-billion-on-cosmetic-plastic-surgery-in-2018.

Arch, J. J., and M. G. Craske. 2006. "Mechanisms of Mindfulness: Emotion Regulation following a Focused Breathing Induction." *Behaviour Research and Therapy* 44 (12): 1849–1858. https://doi.org/10.1016/j.brat.2005.12.007.

Baltazzi, M. 2019. "Why Science Says Helping Others Makes Us Happier." Thrive Global, February 8, 2019. https://thriveglobal.com/stories/why-science-says-helping-others-makes-us-happier/.

Baraz, J., and S. Alexander. 2010. "The Helper's High." Greater Good, February 1, 2010. https://greatergood.berkeley.edu/article/item/the_helpers_high.

Baumeister, R. F., and M. R. Leary. 1995. "The Need to Belong: Desire for Interpersonal Attachments as a Fundamental Human Motivation." *Psychological Bulletin* 117 (3): 497–529. https://pubmed.ncbi.nlm.nih.gov/7777651/.

Biggers, A. 2018. "Endorphins: Effects and How to Boost Them." Medical News Today, February 6, 2018. https://www.medicalnewstoday.com/articles/320839.php.

Blatt, S. J. 1995. "The Destructiveness of Perfectionism: Implications for the Treatment of Depression." *American Psychologist* 50 (12): 1003–1020. https://doi.org/10.1037/0003-066x.50.12.1003.

REFERENCES

Braehler, C., and K. Neff. n.d. "Self-Compassion for PTSD." Accessed June 10, 2021. https://self-compassion.org/wp-content/uploads/2019/09/Braehler .inpress.pdf.

Breines, J. G., M. V. Thoma, D. Gianferante, L. Hanlin, X. Chen, and N. Rohleder. 2014. "Self-Compassion as a Predictor of Interleukin-6 Response to Acute Psychosocial Stress." *Brain, Behavior, and Immunity* 37:109–114. https://doi .org/10.1016/j.bbi.2013.11.006.

Brewster, J. 2021. "More Than One Mass Shooting per Day Has Occurred in 2021." *Forbes*, April 16, 2021. Accessed June 3, 2021. https://www.forbes .com/sites/jackbrewster/2021/04/16/more-than-one-mass-shooting-per -day-has-occurred-in-2021/?sh=54e751a86493.

Brown, B. 2018. "Brené Brown on Joy and Gratitude." Global Leadership Network, November 21, 2018. https://globalleadership.org/articles/leading -yourself/brene-brown-on-joy-and-gratitude/.

Brown, J., and J. Wong. 2017. "How Gratitude Changes You and Your Brain." Greater Good, June 6, 2017. https://greatergood.berkeley.edu/article/ item/how_gratitude_changes_you_and_your_brain#:~:text=%20New %20research%20is%20starting%20to%20explore%20how.

Brown, W. P. 2011. *Ecclesiastes*. Westminster John Knox Press.

Brustein, M. 2015. "Living with FOMO: Tips." drbrustein.com, July 20, 2015. https://www.drbrustein.com/2015/07/living-with-fomo-tips/.

Buddhist Centre. 2019. "Four Noble Truths." https://thebuddhistcentre.com/ text/four-noble-truths.

Burton, L. R. n.d. "The Neuroscience of Gratitude." Wharton Health Care Management Alumni Association. https://www.whartonhealthcare.org/ the_neuroscience_of_gratitude.

Buswell, R. E. 2004. *Encyclopedia of Buddhism*. Macmillan Library Reference.

Carson, S. H., and E. Langer. 2006. "Mindfulness and Self-Acceptance." ResearchGate, March 2006. https://www.researchgate.net/publication/ 226501882_Mindfulness_and_self-acceptance.

REFERENCES

Casale, S., G. Fioravanti, and L. Rugai. 2016. "Grandiose and Vulnerable Narcissists: Who Is at Higher Risk for Social Networking Addiction?" *Cyberpsychology, Behavior, and Social Networking* 19 (8): 510–515. https://doi.org/10.1089/cyber.2016.0189.

CDC. 2020. "Loneliness and Social Isolation Linked to Serious Health Conditions." May 26, 2020. https://www.cdc.gov/aging/publications/features/lonely-older-adults.html.

Chaudhry, S. R., and W. Gossman. 2020. "Biochemistry, Endorphin." NCBI. https://www.ncbi.nlm.nih.gov/books/NBK470306.

Chowdhury, M. R. 2019. "ACT Therapy: The Theory behind Acceptance and Commitment Therapy." PositivePsychology.com, June 30, 2019. https://positivepsychology.com/act-therapy/.

Clear, J. 2018. "How to Start New Habits That Actually Stick." James Clear, November 13, 2018. https://jamesclear.com/three-steps-habit-change.

Cleveland Clinic. 2020. "Why Downtime Is Essential for Brain Health." June 2, 2020. https://health.clevelandclinic.org/why-downtime-is-essential-for-brain-health/.

CMHA National. 2019. "The Importance of Human Connection." October 17, 2019. https://cmha.ca/blogs/the-importance-of-human-connection.

Coelho, P. 1993. *The Alchemist.* HarperOne.

Collins, N. 2018. "How a Neuroscientist Balances Science and Faith." Stanford News, June 21, 2018. https://news.stanford.edu/2018/06/21/neuroscientist-balances-science-faith/.

Daye, C. A., J. B. Webb, and N. Jafari. 2014. "Exploring Self-Compassion as a Refuge against Recalling the Body-Related Shaming of Caregiver Eating Messages on Dimensions of Objectified Body Consciousness in College Women." *Body Image* 11 (4): 547–556. https://doi.org/10.1016/j.bodyim.2014.08.001.

Desbordes, G., L. T. Negi, T. W. W. Pace, B. A. Wallace, C. L. Raison, and E. L. Schwartz. 2012. "Effects of Mindful-Attention and Compassion Meditation

Training on Amygdala Response to Emotional Stimuli in an Ordinary, Non-meditative State." *Frontiers in Human Neuroscience* 6. https://doi.org/10.3389/fnhum.2012.00292.

Diefenbach, S., and L. Christoforakos. 2017. "The Selfie Paradox: Nobody Seems to Like Them Yet Everyone Has Reasons to Take Them: An Exploration of Psychological Functions of Selfies in Self-Presentation." *Frontiers in Psychology* 8. https://doi.org/10.3389/fpsyg.2017.00007.

Diener, E., and M. E. P. Seligman. 2002. "Very Happy People." *Psychological Science* 13 (1): 81–84. https://doi.org/10.1111/1467-9280.00415.

Dixon, T. 2017. "Key Studies: The Effects of Mindfulness and Meditation on the Brain (Desbordes et al. 2012, and Lazar et al. 2005)." IB Psychology, August 20, 2017. https://tinyurl.com/m4a5xaem.

Doyle, G. 2020. *Untamed*. Dial Press.

Duhigg, C. 2014. *Power of Habit: Why We Do What We Do in Life and Business*. Random House.

Finlay-Jones, A. L., C. S. Rees, and R. T. Kane. 2015. "Self-Compassion, Emotion Regulation and Stress among Australian Psychologists: Testing an Emotion Regulation Model of Self-Compassion Using Structural Equation Modeling." *PLOS One* 10 (7): e0133481. https://doi.org/10.1371/journal.pone.0133481.

Ford, B. Q., P. Lam, O. P. John, and I. B. Mauss. 2018. "The Psychological Health Benefits of Accepting Negative Emotions and Thoughts: Laboratory, Diary, and Longitudinal Evidence." *Journal of Personality and Social Psychology* 115 (6): 1075–1092. https://doi.org/10.1037/pspp0000157.

Greater Good Science Center. n.d. "The Science of Gratitude." Accessed June 10, 2021. https://www.templeton.org/wp-content/uploads/2018/05/Gratitude_whitepaper_fnl.pdf.

Griffiths, M. 2018. "Social Media, Selfies, and Addiction." *Psychology Today*. https://www.psychologytoday.com/us/blog/in-excess/201810/social-media-selfies-and-addiction.

REFERENCES

Habits Buzz. 2017. "How Are Habits Formed in the Brain?" October 4, 2017. https://habitsbuzz.com/how-habits-formed-brain/.

———. 2019. "8 Reasons Why You Don't Stick with New Habits (and How to Stick with Them)." September 8, 2019. https://habitsbuzz.com/how-stick -with-new-habits/.

Hammond, C. 2018. "The Anatomy of Loneliness—Who Feels Lonely? The Results of the World's Largest Loneliness Study." BBC, October 2018. https:// www.bbc.co.uk/programmes/articles/2yzhfv4DvqVp5nZyxBD8G23/who -feels-lonely-the-results-of-the-world-s-largest-loneliness-study.

Harvard Health. 2019. "Sleep and Mental Health." March 18, 2019. https://www .health.harvard.edu/newsletter_article/sleep-and-mental-health.

Haynes, T. 2018. "Dopamine, Smartphones & You: A Battle for Your Time." Science in the News, April 30, 2018. http://sitn.hms.harvard.edu/flash/2018/ dopamine-smartphones-battle-time/.

Henderson, R. 2017. "The Science behind Why People Follow the Crowd." *Psychology Today*, May 24, 2017. https://www.psychologytoday.com/us/blog/ after-service/201705/the-science-behind-why-people-follow-the-crowd.

Herbert, J., and L. Brandsma. n.d. "Understanding and Enhancing Psychological Acceptance." University of New England. https://www.une.edu/sites/ default/files/herbertbrandsma_mindfulness.pdf.

Hollis-Walker, L., and K. Colosimo. 2011. "Mindfulness, Self-Compassion, and Happiness in Non-meditators: A Theoretical and Empirical Examination." *Personality and Individual Differences* 50 (2): 222–227. https://doi.org/10 .1016/j.paid.2010.09.033.

Hölzel, B. K., J. Carmody, M. Vangel, C. Congleton, S. M. Yerramsetti, T. Gard, and S. W. Lazar. 2011. "Mindfulness Practice Leads to Increases in Regional Brain Gray Matter Density." *Psychiatry Research: Neuroimaging* 191 (1): 36–43. https://doi.org/10.1016/j.pscychresns.2010.08.006.

Horn, S. 2012. "Singing Changes Your Brain." *Time*, August 16, 2013. https:// ideas.time.com/2013/08/16/singing-changes-your-brain/.

REFERENCES

House, J., K. Landis, and D. Umberson. 1988. "Social Relationships and Health." *Science* 241 (4865): 540–545. https://doi.org/10.1126/science.3399889.

Icahn School of Medicine at Mount Sinai. n.d. "Brain Reward Pathways." https:// neuroscience.mssm.edu/nestler/nidappg/brain_reward_pathways.html.

Keating, S. n.d. "The World's Most Accessible Stress Reliever." BBC. https:// www.bbc.com/future/article/20200518-why-singing-can-make-you-feel -better-in-lockdown.

Kelly, J. n.d. "Indeed Study Shows That Worker Burnout Is at Frighteningly High Levels: Here Is What You Need to Do Now." *Forbes*. Accessed June 5, 2021. https://tinyurl.com/yrxr6zd7.

Kennelly, S. 2012. "What Motivates Kids to Help Others?" Greater Good, June 19, 2012. https://greatergood.berkeley.edu/article/item/what_motivates _kids_to_help_others.

Konrath, S. n.d. "Speaking of Psychology: The Decline of Empathy and the Rise of Narcissism." American Psychological Association. https://www.apa.org/ research/action/speaking-of-psychology/empathy-narcissism.

Konrath, S. H., E. H. O'Brien, and C. Hsing. 2010. "Changes in Dispositional Empathy in American College Students over Time: A Meta-analysis." *Personality and Social Psychology Review* 15 (2): 180–198. https://doi.org/10 .1177/1088868310377395.

Kross, E., M. G. Berman, W. Mischel, E. E. Smith, and T. D. Wager. 2011. "Social Rejection Shares Somatosensory Representations with Physical Pain." *Proceedings of the National Academy of Sciences* 108 (15): 6270–6275. https:// doi.org/10.1073/pnas.1102693108.

Kukk, C. 2017. *The Compassionate Achiever: How Helping Others Fuels Success.* HarperOne.

Lazar, S. W., C. E. Kerr, R. H. Wasserman, J. R. Gray, D. N. Greve, M. T. Treadway, M. McGarvey, B. T. Quinn, J. A. Dusek, H. Benson, S. L. Rauch, C. I. Moore, and B. Fischl. 2005. "Meditation Experience Is Associated with

REFERENCES

Increased Cortical Thickness." *Neuroreport* 16 (17): 1893–1897. https://www
.ncbi.nlm.nih.gov/pmc/articles/PMC1361002/.

Leaf, C. 2020. "I'm a Neuroscientist & Here's Why You Need to Stop 'Milkshake
Thinking.'" MindBodyGreen, October 9, 2020. https://www.mindbodygreen
.com/articles/multitasking-brain-health?fbclid=IwAR12DJGkbQC_jd
-nWxm5aL7nAvw80mJYml9ynHyJ8FI--LiR5AhCerybF0s.

Leonard, A. 2020. "Root to Rise: Tracing Back along the History of Mindfulness." Blinkist, July 31, 2020. https://www.blinkist.com/magazine/posts/
history-of-mindfulness.

Lieberman, D. Z., and M. E. Long. 2019. *The Molecule of More: How a Single
Chemical in Your Brain Drives Love, Sex, and Creativity—and Will Determine the Fate of the Human Race.* BenBella.

Lohmann, R. C. 2015. "Achieving Happiness by Helping Others." *Psychology
Today*, January 29, 2017. https://www.psychologytoday.com/us/blog/teen
-angst/201701/achieving-happiness-helping-others.

Love, S. 2018. "How to Tell If You Have a Dopaminergic Personality." Vice,
August 14, 2018. https://www.vice.com/en/article/d3e53w/theres-a-chemical
-in-your-brain-that-makes-you-want-more.

Luthar, S. S., and C. C. Sexton. 2004. "The High Price of Affluence." *Advances
in Child Development and Behavior* 32:125–162. https://www.ncbi.nlm.nih
.gov/pmc/articles/PMC4358932/.

MacBeth, A., and A. Gumley. 2012. "Exploring Compassion: A Meta-analysis of
the Association between Self-Compassion and Psychopathology." *Clinical
Psychology Review* 32 (6): 545–552. https://doi.org/10.1016/j.cpr.2012.06.003.

Marshall, J. 2019. "Are Religious People Happier, Healthier? Our New Global
Study Explores This Question." Pew Research Center, January 31, 2019.
https://www.pewresearch.org/fact-tank/2019/01/31/are-religious-people
-happier-healthier-our-new-global-study-explores-this-question/.

Martela, F., B. Greve, B. Rothstein, and J. Saari. 2020. "The Nordic Exception-
alism: What Explains Why the Nordic Countries Are Constantly among

REFERENCES

the Happiest in the World." World Happiness Report, March 20, 2020. https://worldhappiness.report/ed/2020/the-nordic-exceptionalism-what -explains-why-the-nordic-countries-are-constantly-among-the-happiest -in-the-world/.

Martino, J., J. Pegg, and E. P. Frates. 2015. "The Connection Prescription: Using the Power of Social Interactions and the Deep Desire for Connectedness to Empower Health and Wellness." *American Journal of Lifestyle Medicine* 11 (6): 466–475. https://doi.org/10.1177/1559827615608788.

Matthews, L. 2017. "What Is Hygge? Everything You Need to Know about the Danish Lifestyle Trend." Country Living, January 6, 2017. https://www .countryliving.com/life/a41187/what-is-hygge-things-to-know-about-the -danish-lifestyle-trend/.

May, A. n.d. "I Wish My Mom's Phone Wasn't Invented, 2nd Grader Writes in School Project." *USA Today*. Accessed June 7, 2021. https://www.usatoday .com/story/tech/nation-now/2018/05/24/2nd-graders-tell-teacher-wish -mom-phone-wasnt-invented/640059002/.

Merriam-Webster. n.d. "FOMO." Accessed October 6, 2021. https://www .merriam-webster.com/dictionary/FOMO.

McDaniel, B. T., and J. S. Radesky. 2017. "Technoference: Parent Distraction with Technology and Associations with Child Behavior Problems." *Child Development* 89 (1): 100–109. https://doi.org/10.1111/cdev.12822.

McKay, B., and K. McKay. 2013. "What Is a Man? The Allegory of the Chariot." Art of Manliness, March 4, 2013. https://www.artofmanliness.com/ articles/what-is-a-man-the-allegory-of-the-chariot/.

McPherson, M., L. Smith-Lovin, and M. E. Brashears. 2006. "Social Isolation in America: Changes in Core Discussion Networks over Two Decades." *American Sociological Review* 71 (3): 353–375. https://doi.org/10.1177/ 000312240607100301.

Merriam-Webster Dictionary. n.d. "Contented." https://www.merriam-webster .com/dictionary/contented.

Mills, J. S., S. Musto, L. Williams, and M. Tiggemann. 2018. "'Selfie' Harm: Effects on Mood and Body Image in Young Women." *Body Image* 27:86–92. https://doi.org/10.1016/j.bodyim.2018.08.007.

Mineo, L. 2017. "Over Nearly 80 Years, Harvard Study Has Been Showing How to Live a Healthy and Happy Life." *Harvard Gazette*, April 11, 2017. https:// news.harvard.edu/gazette/story/2017/04/over-nearly-80-years-harvard -study-has-been-showing-how-to-live-a-healthy-and-happy-life/.

Misiner, D. 2017. "Selfie Paradox: People Want Fewer Selfies on Social Media but Keep Posting Selfies Themselves." CBC, February 21, 2017. https://www.cbc .ca/news/science/selfie-paradox-study-university-of-munich-1.3992182.

Moccia, L., M. Mazza, M. D. Nicola, and L. Janiri. 2018. "The Experience of Pleasure: A Perspective between Neuroscience and Psychoanalysis." *Frontiers in Human Neuroscience* 12 (359). https://doi.org/10.3389/fnhum.2018.00359.

Moll, J., F. Krueger, R. Zahn, M. Pardini, R. de Oliveira-Souza, and J. Grafman. 2006. "Human Fronto-Mesolimbic Networks Guide Decisions about Charitable Donation." *Proceedings of the National Academy of Sciences* 103 (42): 15623–15628. https://doi.org/10.1073/pnas.0604475103.

Monroe, J. 2019. "How to Recognize Loneliness in Teenagers" Newport Academy, January 30, 2019. https://www.newportacademy.com/resources/ mental-health/loneliness-in-teenagers/.

Moulds, J. 2019. "Costa Rica Is One of the World's Happiest Countries. Here's What It Does Differently." World Economic Forum, January 31, 2019. https://www.weforum.org/agenda/2019/01/sun-sea-and-stable-democracy -what-s-the-secret-to-costa-rica-s-success/.

Musick, S. 2021. "Early Treatment for Anorexia Nervosa." Eating Disorder Hope, April 28, 2021. https://www.eatingdisorderhope.com/blog/early -treatment-for-anorexia-nervosa.

National Institute of Mental Health. 2017. "Any Anxiety Disorder." November 2017. https://www.nimh.nih.gov/health/statistics/any-anxiety-disorder .shtml.

REFERENCES

Nazish, N. 2019. "How to De-stress in 5 Minutes or Less, According to a Navy Seal." *Forbes*, May 30, 2019. https://www.forbes.com/sites/nomanazish/2019/05/30/how-to-de-stress-in-5-minutes-or-less-according-to-a-navy-seal/?sh=398590b83046.

NBC News. 2020. "Americans Are the Unhappiest They've Been in 50 Years, Poll Finds." June 16, 2020. https://www.nbcnews.com/politics/politics-news/americans-are-unhappiest-they-ve-been-50-years-poll-finds-n1231153.

Neff, K. D. 2003. "The Development and Validation of a Scale to Measure Self-Compassion." *Self and Identity* 2 (3): 223–250. https://doi.org/10.1080/15298860309027.

———. 2015. *Self-Compassion: Stop Beating Yourself Up and Leave Insecurity Behind*. William Morrow.

Neff, K. D., and C. Germer. 2017. "Self-Compassion and Psychological Well-Being." *Oxford Handbook of Compassion Science*, chap. 27.

Neff, K. D., Y.-P. Hsieh, and K. Dejitterat. 2005. "Self-Compassion, Achievement Goals, and Coping with Academic Failure." *Self and Identity* 4 (3): 263–287. https://doi.org/10.1080/13576500444000317.

Neff, K. D., K. L. Kirkpatrick, and S. S. Rude. 2007. "Self-Compassion and Adaptive Psychological Functioning." *Journal of Research in Personality* 41 (1): 139–154. https://doi.org/10.1016/j.jrp.2006.03.004.

Neff, K. D., K. Pisitsungkagarn, and Y.-P. Hsieh. 2008. "Self-Compassion and Self-Construal in the United States, Thailand, and Taiwan." *Journal of Cross-Cultural Psychology* 39 (3): 267–285. https://doi.org/10.1177/0022022108314544.

Neuroscience News. 2019. "Why Are People Religious? A Cognitive Perspective." January 2, 2019. https://neurosciencenews.com/religion-psychology-cognition-10410/.

Newbergh, A. B. 2019. "Neurotheology: This Is Your Brain on Religion." NPR. https://www.npr.org/2010/12/15/132078267/neurotheology-where-religion-and-science-collide.

REFERENCES

Newman, K. 2016. "Five Science-Backed Strategies to Build Resilience." Greater Good. https://greatergood.berkeley.edu/article/item/five_science_backed _strategies_to_build_resilience.

Ngamaba, K. H. 2018. "Are Religious People Happier Than Non-religious People?" Conversation, February 21, 2018. https://theconversation.com/are -religious-people-happier-than-non-religious-people-87394.

O'Bryon, E. n.d. "Altruism." Greater Good. Accessed June 10, 2021. https:// greatergood.berkeley.edu/topic/altruism.

O'Conner, M. n.d. "The Neuroscience of 'We': How Enhancing Our Connections Can Heal Us." Ornish Lifestyle Medicine. Accessed June 11, 2021. https://www.ornish.com/zine/the-neuroscience-of-we-how-enhancing -our-connections-can-heal-us/.

Oliver, Mary. n.d. "The Summer Day." University of New Mexico. http://www .phys.unm.edu/~tw/fas/yits/archive/oliver_thesummerday.html.

Oppong, T. 2019. "Good Social Relationships Are the Most Consistent Predictor of a Happy Life." Center for Compassion and Altruism Research and Education, October 18, 2019. http://ccare.stanford.edu/press_posts /good-social-relationships-are-the-most-consistent-predictor-of-a -happy-life/.

Ortiz-Ospina, E. 2019. "The Rise of Social Media." Our World in Data, September 18, 2019. https://ourworldindata.org/rise-of-social-media.

Ortiz-Ospina, E., and M. Roser. 2013. "Happiness and Life Satisfaction." Our World in Data. https://ourworldindata.org/happiness-and-life-satisfaction.

Palmer, C. 2021. "Harnessing the Power of Habits." American Psychological Association. https://www.apa.org/monitor/2020/11/career-lab-habits.

Parker, M. 2019. "Honeymoon Hashtag Hell." New York Times, June 19, 2019. https://www.nytimes.com/2019/06/19/fashion/weddings/honeymoon -hashtag-hell.html.

REFERENCES

Parker-Pope, T. 2009. "What Are Friends For? A Longer Life." *New York Times*, April 20, 2009. https://www.nytimes.com/2009/04/21/health/21well.html?_r=1&ref=health.

Patel, A. 2014. "10 Habits of Emotionally Resilient People." MindBodyGreen, May 11, 2014. https://www.mindbodygreen.com/0-13698/10-habits-of-emotionally-resilient-people.html.

Pawlowski, A. 2017. "How to Worry Better." NBC News, May 10, 2017. https://www.nbcnews.com/better/amp/ncna757016.

Perry, B. G. F. 1998. "The Relationship between Faith and Well-Being." *Journal of Religion and Health* 37 (2): 125–136. https://www.jstor.org/stable/27511230?seq=1.

Pew Research Center. n.d. "Happiness & Life Satisfaction." Accessed June 5, 2021. https://www.pewresearch.org/topics/life-satisfaction/.

Phillip, A. 2015. "Addicted to Your Cellphone? These Photos May Make You Uncomfortable." *Washington Post*, October 14, 2015. https://www.washingtonpost.com/news/the-intersect/wp/2015/10/14/addicted-to-your-cellphone-these-photos-may-make-you-uncomfortable/.

Pillay, S. 2016. "Greater Self-Acceptance Improves Emotional Well-Being." *Harvard Health Blog*, May 16, 2016. https://www.health.harvard.edu/blog/greater-self-acceptance-improves-emotional-well-201605169546.

Poulin, M. J. 2014. "Volunteering Predicts Health among Those Who Value Others: Two National Studies." *Health Psychology* 33 (2): 120–129. https://doi.org/10.1037/a0031620.

Poulin, M. J., S. L. Brown, A. J. Dillard, and D. M. Smith. 2013. "Giving to Others and the Association between Stress and Mortality." *American Journal of Public Health* 103:1649–1655. https://doi.org/10.2105/AJPH.2012.300876.

Pounders, K., C. M. Kowalczyk, and K. Stowers. 2016. "Insight into the Motivation of Selfie Postings: Impression Management and Self-Esteem."

European Journal of Marketing 50 (9/10): 1879–1892. https://doi.org/10
.1108/ejm-07-2015-0502.

Powell, A. 2018. "Harvard Researchers Study How Mindfulness May Change
the Brain in Depressed Patients." *Harvard Gazette*, April 9, 2018. https://
news.harvard.edu/gazette/story/2018/04/harvard-researchers-study-how
-mindfulness-may-change-the-brain-in-depressed-patients/.

Pressfield, S. 2003. *The War of Art*. Orion.

Psychology Today. 2018. "Hedonic Treadmill." https://www.psychologytoday
.com/us/basics/hedonic-treadmill.

Quinn, S. 2014. "Religion Is a Sure Route to True Happiness." *Washington Post*,
January 24, 2014. https://www.washingtonpost.com/national/religion/
religion-is-a-sure-route-to-true-happiness/2014/01/23/f6522120-8452-11e3
-bbe5-6a2a3141e3a9_story.html.

Radu, S. 2019. "These Are the World's Happiest Countries." US News & World
Report. https://www.usnews.com/news/best-countries/articles/2019-03-20
/these-are-the-worlds-happiest-countries.

Raes, F. 2010. "Rumination and Worry as Mediators of the Relationship
between Self-Compassion and Depression and Anxiety." *Personality and
Individual Differences* 48 (6): 757–761. https://doi.org/10.1016/j.paid.2010
.01.023.

Robinson, B. E. 2020. "Tara Brach on the Healing Effects of Meditation."
Psychology Today, June 25, 2020. https://www.psychologytoday.com/
us/blog/the-right-mindset/202006/tara-brach-the-healing-effects
-meditation.

Roman, M. W. 2014. "Has 'Be Here Now' Become 'Me Here Now'?" *Issues in
Mental Health Nursing* 35 (11): 814–814. https://doi.org/10.3109/01612840
.2014.954069.

Santi, J. 2017. "The Secret to Happiness Is Helping Others." *Time*. https://time
.com/collection/guide-to-happiness/4070299/secret-to-happiness/.

REFERENCES

Santos, L. 2020. "Episode 6: Dial D for Distracted." *Happiness Lab*, June 1, 2020. https://www.happinesslab.fm/season-2-episodes/episode-6-dial-d -for-distracted.

Schulte, B. 2015. "Harvard Neuroscientist: Meditation Not Only Reduces Stress, Here's How It Changes Your Brain." *Washington Post*, May 26, 2015. https://www.washingtonpost.com/news/inspired-life/wp/2015/05/ 26/harvard-neuroscientist-meditation-not-only-reduces-stress-it-literally -changes-your-brain/.

Seppälä, E. 2012. "Connect to Thrive." *Psychology Today*. https://www .psychologytoday.com/us/blog/feeling-it/201208/connect-thrive.

———. n.d. "Empathy Is on the Decline in This Country. A New Book Describes What We Can Do to Bring It Back." *Washington Post*. https:// www.washingtonpost.com/lifestyle/2019/06/11/empathy-is-decline-this -country-new-book-describes-what-we-can-do-bring-it-back/.

Septien, J. 2019. "Why People with Religious Faith Tend to Sleep Better." Aleteia, January 31, 2019. https://aleteia.org/2019/01/31/why-people-with -religious-faith-tend-to-sleep-better/.

Shankar, A., A. McMunn, J. Banks, and A. Steptoe. 2011. "Loneliness, Social Isolation, and Behavioral and Biological Health Indicators in Older Adults." *Health Psychology* 30 (4): 377–385. https://doi.org/10.1037/a0022826.

Sharma, A., V. Madaan, and F. D. Petty. 2006. "Exercise for Mental Health." *Primary Care Companion to the Journal of Clinical Psychiatry* 8 (2): 106. https://www.ncbi.nlm.nih.gov/pmc/articles/PMC1470658/.

Simons, D. 2010. "The Monkey Business Illusion." Posted April 28, 2010. YouTube video. https://www.youtube.com/watch?v=IGQmdoK_ZfY.

Singer, T., and M. Bolz, eds. n.d. "Compassion—Bridging Practice and Science." Accessed June 10, 2021. http://www.compassion-training.org/en/ online/files/assets/basic-html/index.html#231.

SingleCare Team. 2021. "Eating Disorder Statistics 2021." Checkup, June 3, 2020. https://www.singlecare.com/blog/news/eating-disorder-statistics/.

REFERENCES

Sperling, J. 2020. *The Social Dilemma: Social Media and Your Mental Health.* Mclean Hospital, November 4, 2020. https://www.mcleanhospital.org/essential/it-or-not-social-medias-affecting-your-mental-health.

St. Amour, M. 2020. "Pandemic Increasing Suicidal Ideation." Inside Higher Ed, August 17, 2020. https://www.insidehighered.com/news/2020/08/17/suicidal-ideation-rise-college-aged-adults-due-covid-19-pandemic.

Sternlicht, L., and A. Sternlicht. n.d. "Are Wealthy Children More Susceptible to Drug Addiction? The Psychological Cost of Affluence." Family Addiction Specialist. https://www.familyaddictionspecialist.com/blog/are-wealthy-children-more-susceptible-to-drug-addiction-the-psychological-cost-of-affluence.

Stieg, C. 2019. "How to Stay Committed to Your Goals: Tell Someone More Successful Than You, Says New Study." CNBC, September 5, 2019. https://www.cnbc.com/2019/09/05/why-sharing-goals-with-someone-helps-you-achieve-them.html#:~:text=Researchers%20say%20that%20sharing%20your.

StuffMirror. 2015. "Photographer Removes Smartphones from His Photos to Show How Terribly Addicted We've Become." October 13, 2015. https://www.stuffmirror.com/smartphones-removed-photos/.

Sukel, K. 2019. "In Sync: How Humans Are Hard-Wired for Social Relationships." Dana Foundation, November 13, 2019. https://dana.org/article/in-sync-how-humans-are-hard-wired-for-social-relationships/.

Suttie, J. 2013. "Why Are We So Wired to Connect?" Greater Good, December 2, 2013. https://greatergood.berkeley.edu/article/item/why_are_we_so_wired_to_connect.

———. 2019. "The Mindfulness Skill That Is Crucial for Stress." Greater Good, October 28, 2019. https://greatergood.berkeley.edu/article/item/the_mindfulness_skill_that_is_crucial_for_stress.

———. 2020. "How Does Religion Affect Happiness around the World?" Greater Good, July 13, 2020. https://greatergood.berkeley.edu/article/item/how_does_religion_affect_happiness_around_the_world.

REFERENCES

Taylor, S. 2015. "The Problem with Wanting." *Psychology Today*, July 28, 2015. https://www.psychologytoday.com/us/blog/out-the-darkness/201507/the -problem-wanting.

Tolentino, J. 2019. "The Age of Instagram Face." *New Yorker*, December 12, 2019. https://www.newyorker.com/culture/decade-in-review/the-age-of -instagram-face.

Vahratian, A. 2021. "Symptoms of Anxiety or Depressive Disorder and Use of Mental Health Care among Adults during the COVID-19 Pandemic—United States, August 2020–February 2021." *Morbidity and Mortality Weekly Report* 70. https://doi.org/10.15585/mmwr.mm7013e2.

Vaillant, G. E. 2013. "What Are the Secrets to a Happy Life?" Greater Good, August 6, 2013. https://greatergood.berkeley.edu/article/item/what_are _secrets_to_happy_life.

van der Weiden, A., J. Benjamins, M. Gillebaart, J. F. Ybema, and D. de Ridder. 2020. "How to Form Good Habits? A Longitudinal Field Study on the Role of Self-Control in Habit Formation." *Frontiers in Psychology* 11 (27). https:// doi.org/10.3389/fpsyg.2020.00560.

Villani, D., A. Sorgente, P. Iannello, and A. Antonietti. 2019. "The Role of Spirituality and Religiosity in Subjective Well-Being of Individuals with Different Religious Status." *Frontiers in Psychology* 10. https://doi.org/10.3389/ fpsyg.2019.01525.

Waldinger, R. 2015. "What Makes a Good Life? Lessons from the Longest Study on Happiness." TED Talks video, 12:38. https://www.ted.com/talks/ robert_waldinger_what_makes_a_good_life_lessons_from_the_longest _study_on_happiness?language=en.

Walsh, B. 2017. "Does Spirituality Make You Happy?" *Time*, August 7, 2017. https://time.com/4856978/spirituality-religion-happiness/.

Weinschenk, S. 2019. "The Science of Habits." *Psychology Today*, April 19, 2019. https://www.psychologytoday.com/us/blog/brain-wise/201904/the -science-habits.

REFERENCES

Weller, C. 2018. "Bill Gates and Steve Jobs Raised Their Kids Tech-Free—and It Should've Been a Red Flag." Business Insider, January 10, 2018. https://www.businessinsider.com/screen-time-limits-bill-gates-steve-jobs-red-flag-2017-10.

White, T. 2010. "Love Takes Up Where Pain Leaves Off, Brain Study Shows." News Center, October 13, 2010. https://med.stanford.edu/news/all-news/2010/10/love-takes-up-where-pain-leaves-off-brain-study-shows.html.

Wood, A., J. Linley, and A. Linley. 2020. "Gratitude—Parent of All Virtues." Psychologist. https://thepsychologist.bps.org.uk/volume-20/edition-1/gratitude-parent-all-virtues.

World Happiness Report. 2019. "The Sad State of Happiness in the United States and the Role of Digital Media." March 20, 2019. https://worldhappiness.report/ed/2019/the-sad-state-of-happiness-in-the-united-states-and-the-role-of-digital-media/.

Woronko, M. 2015. "Addiction to Selfies: A Mental Disorder?" Lifehack, February 10, 2015. https://www.lifehack.org/articles/communication/addiction-selfies-mental-disorder.html.